ATHLETIC DEVELOPMENT

The Art & Science
of Functional Sports Conditioning

ATHLETIC DEVELOPMENT

The Art & Science
of Functional Sports Conditioning

Vern Gambetta

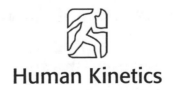

Human Kinetics

Library of Congress Cataloging-in-Publication Data

Gambetta, Vern.
 Athletic development : the art & science of functional sports conditioning / Vern Gambetta.
   p. cm.
 Includes bibliographical references and index.
 ISBN-13: 978-0-7360-5100-2 (soft cover)
 ISBN-10: 0-7360-5100-7 (soft cover)
 1. Physical education and training. I. Title.
 GV341.G323 2007
 613.7--dc22

                                2006026774

ISBN-10: 0-7360-5100-7
ISBN-13: 978-0-7360-5100-2

Developmental Editor: Heather Healy; **Assistant Editor:** Christine Horger; **Copyeditor:** Jan Feeney; **Proofreader:** Bethany Bentley; **Indexers:** Robert and Cynthia Swanson; **Permission Manager:** Carly Breeding; **Graphic Designer:** Fred Starbird; **Graphic Artist:** Francine Hamerski; **Photo Manager:** Brenda Williams; **Cover Designer:** Keith Blomberg; **Photographer (cover):** Tom Roberts; **Photographer (interior):** Photos on pages 5, 29, 103, and 151 © Human Kinetics, all other photos by Brenda Williams unless otherwise noted; **Art Manager:** Kelly Hendren; **Illustrator:** Jason McAlexander; **Printer:** United Graphics

Human Kinetics books are available at special discounts for bulk purchase. Special editions or book excerpts can also be created to specification. For details, contact the Special Sales Manager at Human Kinetics.

Printed in the United States of America   10

The paper in this book is certified under a sustainable forestry program.

Human Kinetics
Web site: www.HumanKinetics.com

United States: Human Kinetics, P.O. Box 5076, Champaign, IL 61825-5076
800-747-4457
email: humank@hkusa.com

Canada: Human Kinetics, 475 Devonshire Road Unit 100, Windsor, ON N8Y 2L5
800-465-7301 (in Canada only)
email: info@hkcanada.com

Europe: Human Kinetics, 107 Bradford Road, Stanningley, Leeds LS28 6 AT, United Kingdom
+44 (0) 113 255 5665
email: hk@hkeurope.com

Australia: Human Kinetics, 57A Price Avenue, Lower Mitcham, South Australia 5062
08 8372 0999
e-mail: info@hkaustralia.com

New Zealand: Human Kinetics, P.O. Box 80, Torrens Park, South Australia 5062
0800 222 062
e-mail: info@hknewzealand.com

To my family, my wife, Melissa, my toughest critic but the person who is always there for support. Without her none of this would have been possible. To my children, Curt and Kristen, who are a parent's dream. Their achievements continue to inspire me.

Contents

Foreword

Imagine, if you will, a system of continual progress toward improvement. This system is of a social nature, for it has examined the effects of location in the world, political climate, economic status, and importance to the community. This system is of a scientific nature, for it has examined the effects of physics, biology, anatomy, physiology, and mathematical principles that help shed light on how things can work. This system is of a competitive nature; it forever realizes that constant adjustments are necessary for achieving and maintaining success. Above all, this system is of a human nature; it understands that no person is perfect, no plan perfect, and no system perfect. The system maintains a continual use of checks and balances: self-check, self-critique, evaluate, reevaluate, and then move forward, onward, and upward.

Now imagine a scenario that has you send someone out into the world to gather information. He or she would have to be someone with a critical eye for quality information. We must imagine someone who has an intense thirst for knowledge in any area that has an effect on our particular field or endeavor. This person will continually gather information, store it, and refer to it for the purposes of raising levels of understanding. Imagine this person as someone who spans the globe to not only gather but bounce information off of different cultures, societies, programs, and activities. This person not only collects this information but uses it, applies it, evaluates it, and rates its usefulness to others. This person asks the tough questions in an attempt to truly understand the whys, whens, whos, and hows.

Finally, imagine if this person could compile and condense this wealth of information into a refined, simplified reservoir of information. This person then disperses the information, blending the world's best minds in the field.

With Vern Gambetta and the text that he has written in the following pages, you do not need to imagine any longer. Having known Vern for three decades, I can assure you that the information you are about to read represents a true quest toward improvement in the world of athleticism. His quest has spanned many parts of the world, cultures, and training systems and culminated in a body of information that only the Internet could match. What the Internet won't do is give you the deciphered version. The information in these chapters has been researched, used and observed, and applied in familiar contexts we can understand.

The most important point that can be made about what lies in the following pages is that it truly is a highly thought out and planned out series of training. To many of us, training for sport and athleticism is like a religion. There is a spiritual nature to the process of learning about and obtaining athletic fitness, and to the reading of the signs or signals that tell us to push on, back off, or find balance in the work. Similar to other religions, there can be many differences in approach, style, and beliefs, though there is often a common set of objectives or outcomes at the core. The exciting part is that in the course of examining the information Vern has set forth, you will discover the systematic approaches that you need in order to read the signs and walk the path toward more intelligent and productive training.

James C. Radcliffe
Head Strength and Conditioning Coach
University of Oregon

Acknowledgments

This book is really written by all of those who have influenced me throughout my life. Preparing these acknowledgments made me realize how fortunate and blessed I have been. I would like to thank everyone who has helped directly and indirectly throughout my career. I have been very privileged to be associated with so many great people that I am not sure where to begin. The best place to start is with the athletes: The La Cumbre Junior High School track and cross country teams and the Santa Barbara High boys' and girls' track and cross country teams. I hope you all learned as much from me as I did from you. Some of my fondest memories are from those years and those athletes. The men's track team at Stanford 1973-74, the Cal Berkeley women's track and cross country teams, the White Sox, the Tampa Bay Mutiny, and my decathletes Scott Daniels and Steve Odgers.

I have been very fortunate to have been exposed to outstanding teachers and mentors. Mr. Charles Kuehl, my high school basketball coach and European History teacher, who forced me to grow up. He was my first exposure to real coaching. Red Estes who got me into coaching track and field. Sherm Button, who taught me the fundamentals of strength training and took an interest in what I was doing. Marshall Clark, who allowed me to get my foot in the door in college coaching and taught me the necessity of patience and humility. Bill Crow, the first head coach I worked for who walked and talked softly but carried a big stick. Gary Gray, who solidified my ideas about functional training. Al Goldis, my boss with the White Sox, who gave me the chance to innovate in pro baseball. Joe Vigil, the consummate professional, who taught me never to lower my expectations, because he would not allow it. Jimmy Radcliffe, who wrote the foreword, is the best athletic development coach I know. Gary Winckler, simply the best coach I know and a great friend. John Larralde, a loyal and true friend. Steve Myrland, a great friend who has been a continual source of ideas and great sounding board over the years. Kevin McGill, whose prodding and encouragement forced me to get this book done. Last but not least, my parents, who have been my inspiration throughout my life. I wish they were alive to read this. Their encouragement and sacrifice allowed me to get an education and achieve anything I have achieved in my life. Thanks, Mom and Dad.

Elements of a Training System

part I

A Functional Conditioning Framework

When I look at sports from a perspective of movement, not one of skill, I see beauty and flow. All throws look fundamentally the same; all jumps look the same; acceleration, regardless of the sport, looks the same. The only things that change are the implement, the surface, and the uniform in the sport.

When I coach, I look for the commonalities in movements and train those commonalities. All sports involve some of these movements: running, jumping, throwing, pushing, pulling, reaching, lifting, bending, extending, stopping, and starting. When I set out to design and implement a conditioning program, I am aware of all these movements and how they efficiently blend and flow into athletic skill.

To design an effective training program, you need to train fundamental movement skills before training specific sport skills. This is contrary to the typical approach in which sport skill is taught early and the sport is used as conditioning. Specific sport skill is a blend of a series of movements into the whole, which is the objective. Start with a vision of how you want the athlete to look at the end of the training program, and then break it down into progressive parts to arrive at that point, but never lose sight of the whole. The ultimate result is a functional training program.

Functional training has taken many forms as it has evolved. No one form is correct or incorrect; it is just important to remember the principles of functional training as defined in this book and to use them as evaluative criteria. Functional training involves more than working on unstable surfaces and using stability balls and stretch cords. It encompasses a range of methods and applications that aid in the transfer of training to competition. Because functional training is evolving, it is open to innovation.

Function employs an integrated (as opposed to isolated) approach. It involves movement of multiple body parts, and the movement involves multiple planes. This simple definition has incredibly complex applications that are developed throughout the rest of this book. It is not a matter of functional or nonfunctional; rather it is an understanding of how functional a particular movement or exercise is relative to the training objective. If an athlete is working to improve strength for running, and the exercises he is doing involve seated or prone positions, then they are not very functional with respect to the goal of improving strength for running. On the other hand, those exercises would be functional for a rower who performs tasks in a seated position.

Movements that are less functional are isolated, repetitive movements. Examples are the leg extension and leg curl. These exercises repeat themselves, and they are an end in themselves. Contrast this to the lunge, which is progressive and can lead to many variations. The body is a linked system, and movement involves the timing of the movement of the links of the kinetic chain. It is helpful to visualize the process as total-chain training, moving from toenails to fingernails. The outcome is functional sports training, which incorporates a global-systems approach to training and rehabilitation. *Functional training* can be a misleading term because all movement is functional. The distinction must be made regarding functionality of the exercise or drill relative to the movements in the sport. To address movement relative to the sport, think of placing movements on a continuum of function. (See figure 1.1.)

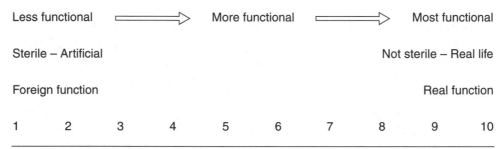

Figure 1.1 Continuum of function.

Use the continuum of function to conceptually organize the evaluation of exercises or training methods. If you spend too much time on the left of the continuum, the work will not transfer as rapidly as work done on the right of the continuum. Obviously in rating a training task or activity on the continuum of function, the activity itself is a 10. Work back from there. A good training program will incorporate activities moving along the continuum with a concentration of work on the right. The following are evaluative criteria for placement on the continuum of function:

- Is the movement or exercise in one plane or is it in multiple planes?
- Is the movement isolated at one joint, or does it involve multiple joints?
- Is the speed of the movement as fast as can be controlled?
- Is the objective of the exercise to train a skill needed for the sport?
- Is conditioning the objective of the exercise?

Training for function is training with variety for a specific purpose. Functional training taps into the wisdom of the body. So learn to observe the body's functioning in the context of the movement so that training will be functional.

THE FUNCTIONAL PATH

In my experience as a coach, particularly as a conditioning coach, following the functional path has at times been frustrating but ultimately a satisfying experience. Initially I found there were not many sources of information. But the farther I traveled down the path, the more I found signs that many people had been there before. I would see a concept here and a training method there. I would hear a presentation or read an article. All of these methods were on the track, but there was no unified direction. I realized that in order for success to occur in athletic development, commonalities had to occur.

The most successful people I encountered along the path really knew and understood movement. They could sense and feel and articulate how the body moved. Most important, they understood how the body moved efficiently. Some of these people were coaches; some were athletes, artists, dancers, physical therapists, or sport scientists. What they all had in common was a feeling for the body as a unit, a kinetic chain, where movement was more than just individual muscles contracting and relaxing. They understood that each link in the chain had a specific role to play, that each link is part of an integrated whole, resulting in efficient flowing movement. If there was a problem somewhere in the chain, they could look at the links above or below the problem to determine the cause.

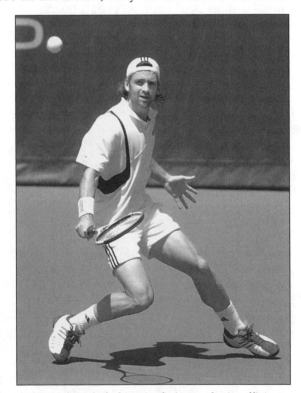

I had the most success as a coach when I emphasized training the kinetic chain. I noticed that when I spent too much time on one part of the chain (one link), I would have trouble getting that part to work smoothly with its partners in the whole chain. That is essentially how I arrived at the functional approach. Training the whole system, understanding the interrelationship and interdependency of the links, is what function is about. It is free flowing, not segmented. It is rhythmic, not jumpy.

Just as all movement is functional and all training is good, the question is *how* good. The more functional

Training the whole kinetic chain results in efficient flowing movement.

(function being relative to the activity or sport a person is training for), the more effective the training. It took me a while to realize that just because an athlete could "feel the burn" in training, that did not mean that it was good training. Just because an athlete was "ripped" did not mean that that muscle mass would transfer to performance. I look at a simple criterion: If I am getting too far away from fundamental movement, then what I am doing is not highly functional, and it won't transfer. There is an adage in coaching: You are what you train to be. If you train to be slow, you will be slow. If you train to be explosive, you will be explosive.

PHILOSOPHY OF FUNCTIONAL TRAINING

A well-grounded philosophy is the cornerstone on which everything else is built. That is especially true in sports conditioning. A sound philosophy is required for effective methods and consistent, positive results. This was impressed on me early in my coaching career through study, observation, and interaction with great coaches. Bill Bowerman, renowned track and field coach at the University of Oregon, was the featured speaker at the first coaching clinic I ever attended. His pragmatic, eclectic, and versatile philosophy and his desire to find a better way to train his athletes were evident throughout his presentation. He had a clearly defined system that he adapted to fit the needs of individual athletes. And it was clear that he believed in and practiced everything he presented. Above all, he was a big-picture thinker.

Bowerman's presentation left an indelible impression on me. Every successful coach I have met and observed since then has a philosophy that clearly guides everything he or she does. Conversely, the unsuccessful coaches either did not have a defined philosophy or frequently changed philosophies. Once established, these foundational beliefs do not change.

My coaching philosophy can be summed up by this quote from George Bernard Shaw: "Some see things as they are and ask why. Others dream things that never were and ask why not." A logical extension of this quote is the power of the question. Learning to ask the key questions is essential to success. Without the power of the question, there is no possibility of innovation or change. You must recognize that change is a constant if you want to get better and to get the athletes you work with to function better. These are the key questions you must continually ask yourself and the athletes you work with:

- Why are you doing what you are doing?
- How are you actually going to do it?
- What specifically are you going to do?
- When are you going to do it?

Answering those questions will enable you to design the most effective training programs as well as be the best coach you can be. The power of the question leads to the concept of flexible thinking, which will enable you to take the ideas about training presented in the following chapters and adapt them to virtually any situation. Dave Hemery, 1968 Olympic champion in the 400-meter hurdles, said, "Flexible thinking, lateral thinking, openness to new ideas, and a willingness to experiment should be in all our minds. Change seems to be the only constant in life, so we ought to try to make ourselves and the things we come in contact with change for the better." Because change is constant, coaches must learn to manage change. That will be essential to success.

From both a philosophical and practical viewpoint, you must recognize the importance of basics. Know the fundamental movements. You are the coach of people, not of sport. In that light, you must coach the whole person. Coaching is not something you do *to* the athlete; it is something you do in cooperation *with* the athlete. It is a partnership. Never lose sight of the concept of the 24-hour athlete. The athletes you work with train for 2 to 4 hours a day. It is a fundamentally unbalanced equation because the other 20 to 22 hours have more of an impact on the athlete's success or failure in the chosen sport than the training time. It is easy to fall into the trap of training, not coaching. Training is paying attention only to the actual workout: manipulation of sets, reps, heart rates, maximum lifts. Coaching, on the other hand, is developing the whole person mentally, physically, and socially. It is working closely with the athletes to define their goals and teach them how to achieve their goals. Coaching is a creative process that takes imagination and enthusiasm. Coaching empowers the athlete to take a degree of responsibility for his or her actions. As the athlete's career progresses, the athlete should assume a greater degree of responsibility so that you, the coach, assume more of an advisory capacity. Frank Dick, former chief coach of athletics in Great Britain, put it best when he said that during the course of an athlete's career, the coach's role evolves from that of a guiding light to a mirror. Coaching, like parenting, teaching, and managing, provides the roots to grow and the wings to fly.

Ultimately a coach is a teacher. Teaching is communicating, and communication is the key to effective coaching. Communication has the dimensions of both sending and receiving. Coaches, by nature, tend to be good at sending but not always as good at receiving. To be effective, you must cultivate both dimensions of communication. Learn to listen as well as speak. Sometimes it is as simple as being there to support the athlete; words are not always the answer.

The pursuit of excellence has its own rewards. Winning medals and championships is an outcome that is a logical extension of the process. If coaches were judged entirely on wins and losses, there would not be very many successful coaches. It is just as important to enjoy the journey as it is to enjoy the destination. The challenge of learning what it takes to help new athletes or teams achieve their potential is the real joy of coaching. The rings, banners, and trophies are all a bonus.

Each athlete is unique and will present a unique challenge. Therefore, you will need to adjust without compromising your core beliefs. I have coached two athletes of the same age, event, and performance level. But each of them has needed very different training programs to achieve the same result. It took me many years of coaching to realize that everyone progresses at different rates and brings different qualities to respective events and sports. This is a unique challenge, but it is not insurmountable.

No matter how good an athlete is, that athlete can always get better. Every great athlete and coach whom I have worked with was always striving to get better. Carlton Fisk, Hall of Fame catcher, at the end of his career at age 44, was always working extra to improve his game. Michael Jordan, as good as he was, always worked to improve some aspect of his game in every off-season. To watch Larry Bird run a mile three hours before game time and make 200 shots before each game underscored what the best do to get better. Never be complacent. Even if you are the best, you can get better. I am continually amazed by Dr. Joe Vigil, one of the premier track and field coaches in the world, and his insatiable appetite for knowledge. Even though he has a PhD in exercise physiology and several master's degrees, he is always working to increase his knowledge base.

Observing and working with successful people led me to define my mission statement as "training the best to be better" through education and specialized high-performance training. This is accomplished by building the complete athlete or, if the athlete is injured, by rebuilding the complete athlete through a systematic, progressive approach to the total conditioning process.

Historian Arnold Toynbee once said, "Those who cannot remember the past are condemned to repeat it." It is easy to lose sight of what has gone before us. It is important to understand the historical context of the current training methods and ideas. Very little is new. We all stand on the shoulders of giants. We must recognize, acknowledge, and honor those who have gone before us, those who have blazed the functional path so that we may more easily follow. Training modes such as the medicine ball, Indian clubs, still rings, and dumbbells were used extensively in physical education and training in the late 1800s and the early 20th century. Periodization and plyometrics are not new. Since we have rediscovered them, we have a better understanding of their application and role in the big picture of training.

THE ART AND SCIENCE OF COACHING

Coaching is both an art and a science. This is a careful blend, not an either–or proposition. In today's world of rapid change and scientific advances, it is easy to get caught up in the science and minimize the art. Coaching practice should be rooted in science, but you should also have a good experiential base to help athletes achieve their potential.

Everything you do must be based on sound principles. Keep accurate and detailed records so that you can look retrospectively at why something succeeded or why it failed. George Johnson, in his book *Fire in the Mind* (1996, p. 5) put it quite well: "Science is the search for neat predictable curves, compact ways of summarizing the data. But there is danger that curves we see are illusory, like pictures of animals in the clouds. As we draw our self-propelling arcs, some points will inevitably lie outside the line—those that must be dismissed as random error or noise. So we are left with a gnawing dissatisfaction: Are we missing something? If we looked at the points harder, graphed them a different way, would a more elegant order emerge?" This can also help lead the sport scientist to solve practical coaching problems. Once again, as a coach you have to keep in mind the power of the question. You have to be able to ask the sport scientist questions that will direct research into applied areas that will give information that you can use. This is perhaps the biggest change that I have seen during my coaching career. When I started in 1969, there was a huge gap between the sport scientist and the coach. Today there are many sport scientists who speak the language of coaching and are producing great applied research.

For me, the formula for success is relatively simple in concept but complex in application. The formula is 3M + 3P = success. The three Ms are as follows: It must be manageable; by that it must be accomplished in the context of the personnel, facilities, time, and equipment available. It must be measurable; you must be able to see and quantify the results of the training program. It must be motivational; it must be something that you and the athlete look forward to doing. The three Ps are as follows: Everything you do must be practical; it cannot be so complex or require so much time that it cannot be done. It must be personal; it must be adapted to fit the individual needs of each athlete you are working with as well as your individual needs as a coach. It must be proactive; there must be a plan that anticipates the obstacles and adjusts accordingly. Training will produce measurable results. Failing to train will also produce a measurable result. The training process is cumulative.

As a coach, you are always faced with choices. You can take the comfortable route and do what you have always done—follow the crowd, yield to conventional wisdom. This approach does not require any risk, but it eventually produces long-term stagnation. On the other hand, innovation requires risk that often does not result in short-term gain. The innovators use conventional wisdom as a starting point and proceed from there. It is not always comfortable to innovate, but it keeps you involved and alert. It is more than change for the sake of change; it is purposeful change based on sound principles. Have the resolve to design the best program possible. Have the confidence to teach it well and the patience to implement the program and wait for the results. Attend to the details.

COACHING FOR PROPER CONDITIONING

We have cultural, physical, educational, and economic obstacles that coaches from past generations did not have to contend with. Today's society is much more sedentary than previous generations were. That, coupled with an increased intake of food, has resulted in rising rates of obesity. We tend to focus on results rather than appreciate the process. Failure has a social price tag attached to it. Boys will gladly demonstrate proficiency but will often quit before having to reveal deficiency. Girls often fear success if it places them apart from others. Girls must try to resolve the conflict of working to be strong, fit, and fast in a social order that offers few rewards for these qualities in women.

In the context of the athletic arena, we play to train rather than train to play. We specialize before we develop athleticism and competitive maturity. We emphasize game skills before and often to the exclusion of fundamental movement skills. We evaluate before we teach (always trying to find the next prodigy). In training and competition, we value quantity over quality. We are forced into a one-size-fits-all model of drills and exercises, even though one size never does fit all. Play has disappeared. If practice is not organized and there is no coach present, there is no practice. We prefer to watch rather than participate. More is considered better in training. Free play is no longer part of the developmental process. It has been supplanted by structured practices closely supervised by adults. Despite the highly organized nature of youth sport, there seems to be little or no understanding of the needs and desires of young athletes.

I certainly did not have to cope with much of this when I began coaching in 1969, but these challenges are a reality today. Despite these obstacles, there are definite strategies for success. You must know yourself and your strengths and weaknesses as a coach. Know the body and how it responds to training. Learn to see movement better. Great coaches have a great eye. They have cultivated the art of pattern recognition. You must be able to evaluate movement in order to improve it. One size never fits all, but never base a training plan on the lowest common denominator. Set the standards high, and observe what happens. Make things relevant. Make training competitive and keep score.

Be creative. Build movement and drill progressions in which game skills and tactics are included. Learn what you don't know, and do not be limited by what you do know. Create a resource library for yourself and for fellow coaches and parents. Make use of the resources you already have. Knowledge is power; you can never know too much. Beware of mindless rather than mindful preparation. Know the athletes and how they respond to coaching, criticism, praise, competition, losing, and winning. How do the athletes respond physically to training, skill work, recovery, rest, travel, and fatigue? Above all, how do they respond to you as a coach? Specialize in being a generalist so that you can connect and synthesize the information into a coherent whole. Heed the words of Albert Einstein: "Everything should be made as simple as possible, but simpler."

Coaching Creativity

Every composer starts with the same notes. Every author starts with the same alphabet. All artists start with the same palette of basic colors. Why aren't there more Beethovens, Hemingways, and Rembrandts? The answer is genius and the creative process. At the heart of coaching is the creative process. The coach is no different from the composer or the artist. The coach's palette is the human body expressed through movement.

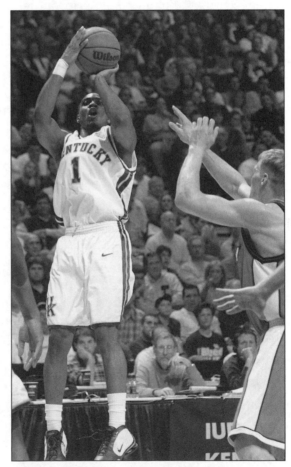

The creative process is not a linear process. The steps in this process are easily adapted to the coaching environment. There is a Buddhist saying that is particularly appropriate: "You don't need to see different things, but rather to see things differently." The more you watch a movement or an activity, the more you tend to overlook the nuances that make the movement unique.

Strive to see common activities in a new way to observe the nuances of an athlete's movement.
© Charles Small/SportsChrome

Look for differences and patterns in each athlete's movement. Change the vantage point. If you always watch from the side, change sides or move to the back. A whole new vista will open up. Look for the flow and feel the rhythm. That will allow you to see the same things differently.

As the training programs for the various sports are designed and implemented, certain commonalities between sports are apparent. In fact, once you get away from the nuances of the sport and focus on the movements, there will be more similarities than differences. Look carefully for commonalities between sports before looking for differences. Once you find commonalties, find as many ways to link them. You will find more commonalities than you thought were possible. And by looking for commonalities, you will see the differences.

The system of sport classification discussed in chapter 3 will point you in the right direction by dictating the selection of the training methods. In selecting exercises for training, you may have similar exercises or even the same exercises, but you can perform them differently (at a different tempo, with or without resistance) to adapt the exercises to the respective sport. The message is that it is more than an exercise; it is the context in which the exercise is applied that ultimately will matter the most.

Use creativity in building an effective training program. Incorporating the principles and concepts from the upcoming chapters is a step-by-step process. Once you have analyzed and classified the sport, start with a clear image of the finished product. What should an athlete look like and be able to accomplish when the training program is completed? This must be articulated in terms that everyone can understand and relate to. Without the end in sight, it is difficult to determine the appropriate steps to achieve that product.

How much time is available to train outside of actual technical and tactical sport practice? How much more time is needed? Reconcile the two, or else the training program will be constantly conflicted. There is no substitute for time, but what you do with the time is most important. About 30 to 40 minutes a day during the in-season is more than enough time, and 75 to 90 minutes in the noncompetitive phase is sufficient to get the job done. Also consider the amount of time in terms of weeks. To achieve any kind of significant changes, a program must be at least six weeks in length. It is unrealistic to expect any significant progress in less time unless the athlete is a rank beginner. Do not try to design and implement crash programs because they usually do crash. Be realistic in the time frame to allow the program to work; keep in mind the time needed for adaptation of various motor qualities. Once you have clearly established the time frame, decide on the actual structure of the plan. Chapter 6 will help you determine goals for each training block in specific and measurable terms. Then determine themes based on the goals. Remember that the plan must be dynamic. It also must be a collaborative process.

Ultimately the plan will be determined by the timing and sequence of the appropriate training stimulus. It is not as much about what is done as it is about when and how it is done. For example, a session of heavy squats for a sprinter in track and field can be an appropriate workout for a general preparation block of training but would be counterproductive in a competition block. Anyone can work, but productive work must have a purpose and direction. Work is easy. Directing the work is difficult. The interaction of the various components to allow proper stress and adequate time for adaptation is the secret to effective training. Carefully consider the following:

- **Sequence** refers to the general categories of work. You know that it is counterproductive to train absolute strength and aerobic endurance in the same training block or try to emphasize both equally in the same training block.

- **Order** refers to the actual exercises. There is an optimal order in training various qualities depending on the emphasis in training.

- **Timing** refers to when the stress is applied. This involves applying the principles of planned performance covered in chapter 5.

Coaching Strategies

There are no quick fixes or shortcuts, even with younger athletes; it is a long-term process. With young developing athletes, keep it *fun*damental. Biological age is much more important than chronological age. The *can do* and *want to do* are quite different; do not be in a hurry. With female athletes, recognize the differences and coach the differences. With master's athletes, training is an accumulation of previous work, both positive and negative. With elite athletes, recognize what got them to that level and build on that. Despite the fact that a chapter of the book is devoted to recovery, remember that recovery is important only if the training has been stressful enough to necessitate recovery. So carefully look at the proportion of work to rest that will allow optimal time for adaptation.

Attention to detail and good effort will produce optimal results in the long term. Nick Green, one of the famous Australian "Oarsome Foursome" rowers who won the gold medal in the 1996 Olympics, summed it up quite well: "For us, it was definitely quality. A simple scenario: We race over two kilometers and take about 220 to 240 strokes per race. Our aim in training was to work on various aspects of our preparation so that on race day, our boat would go half an inch faster per stroke than every stroke of our opposition. We knew that we weren't the biggest or strongest guys in the competition, so we had to look at other ways of generating boat speed. This is a sport that is built on strength and endurance. So our focus was on our quality and efficiency of movement, particularly in our technique. If you look at the margin we won by in Atlanta, it equated to roughly two-thirds of a second per stroke quicker than the second boat."

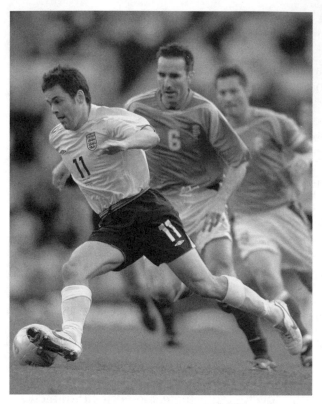

Winning everyday workouts leads to success in the competitive arena.

© Empics

Wayne Goldsmith presents a good paradigm when looking at the parameters of a successful sport development program. He recommends that the program be athlete centered, coach driven, and administratively supported. It's simply common sense. The program should be about the athletes and how you as a coach can make the athletes better. That requires committed and educated coaches who have the support of administration.

The actual workout and management of training is where the rubber meets the road. This is where the goal is simple and straightforward: to "win the workout." You must do this consistently before you can win a competition. An accumulation of workout wins leads to success in the competitive arena. To consistently win the workout, you must control these essential elements: personnel, facilities, equipment, and a contingency plan. Keep in mind that the laws of physiology and physics are not suspended during the workout.

To consistently win the workout, consider training to your strengths. Training to your strengths is certainly not a new idea but in many ways it runs contrary to the way most coaches think. There is something about coaches and coaching that leads coaches to do the opposite—to train the weaknesses. Before you focus on what athletes cannot do, find out everything they can do. What are their strengths? How do they use their strengths at the present time? Is an inordinate amount of emphasis given to training to improve weaknesses to the exclusion of the strengths?

With young developing athletes, ask the obvious question: Are they in the correct event or even in the right sport? Sometimes what is perceived as a weakness in one event will be a strength in another sport. Find the talent that suits the event; do not try to make athletes what they are not. Each athlete's strengths are unique and personal. The more that you can help athletes explore their strengths, the more solid they will be on the training.

Learn to manage the weaknesses. To begin to deal with the weakness, you and the athletes first need to identify it. Is it something that is holding an athlete back from being significantly better? One approach is to let the strengths overwhelm the weakness. Athletes should ask themselves whether it is really their weaknesses that are defeating or whether they are not completely exploiting their strengths. To truly be a strength, an athlete must be able to do it consistently. Athletes should not take their strengths for granted; they need to learn them and appreciate them.

Stay objective, because losing objectivity will distort both success and failure. The curve of progression should be undulating and rising, not a roller-coaster ride. Clear the path. Remove obstacles that could interfere with achievement of training objectives. Focus, focus, and focus more to stay on the functional path. Inconsistent training does not produce consistent, measurable performance results. The following are specific criteria for focused exercise selection:

- Movement must involve multiple joints.
- Movement must involve multiple planes.
- Training should be proprioceptively demanding.
- Train at a speed and amplitude of movement that the athlete can control.
- Identify the training priorities.
- Choose the methods to achieve those priorities.
- Select the means of training.
- Develop a menu of drills, exercises, and specific training modules.
- Choose appropriate tests and evaluation methods to measure results.

You see what you are trained to see. Learn to see with different eyes. Broaden the perspective. Work to eliminate bias. Always keep the big picture in mind. Once the big picture is lost, it is easy to lose control of the whole process. Big-picture thinking demands that everything be kept in context. As in a symphony, all sections must be in harmony. No global motor quality can stand alone; it must be supported by the other qualities to produce results. Trying to work on a component in isolation will ultimately limit the ability to develop that quality to its fullest extent. All qualities are related and in many respects interdependent. Take full advantage of that interdependence to develop the optimal training program.

Beware of those who teach or preach one way. Some paths to functional performance are clear and direct and some paths are narrow, unpaved, and strewn with obstacles. Use the information presented in this book to guide you regardless of the condition of the path. The deeper your understanding of functional training, the fewer tools you will actually use. The tools you do use will be more specific and effective. A clear understanding of the factors of movement discussed in chapter 2, as well as the principles of functional training will allow more effective choice of the appropriate tools for the specific situation.

There are different approaches to planning, designing, and implementing a training program. The qualitative (right-brain) approach tends to lean toward broad brush strokes, trends, and themes. The quantitative (left-brain) approach tends to be more mathematical, logical, and exact. Both work well. The choice of approach is dictated by your philosophy, personality, and background. Certainly the best approach is a combination. There are some basic coaching dos and don'ts:

- Evaluate.
- Plan.
- Clearly define objectives.
- Determine means and methods to reach those objectives.
- Create an environment where champions are inevitable.
- Work with purpose and direction.
- Know your strengths and weaknesses as a coach.
- Define yourself; do not let others define you.
- Design training sessions that foster and encourage discovery. Do not create robots.
- Beware of the "monkey see, monkey do" syndrome. Just because the champion does it does not mean that it is appropriate training for the athletes you are working with. They may be succeeding in spite of, not because of, the training.
- Teach and encourage routine first.
- Don't get caught in the density trap. Everything does not have to be done in seven days.
- Don't mix methods within a workout. Each workout should have a neural emphasis or metabolic emphasis, but not both.
- Don't lose sight of the fact that training is a means to an end, not an end in itself. Training is preparing to compete.

Role of the Athletic Development Coach

The state of the profession is in flux. There is no consensus on the definition of strength and conditioning or on the role of a strength and conditioning coach. I have seen many strength coaches who never leave the weight room because they view themselves as just that—strength coaches. To achieve consensus we must define the field; currently it is all over the map. There needs to be consistent direction and purpose. Coaching is not personal training, although personal attention is certainly part of coaching. At present the field is called strength and conditioning, a field that evolved out of American football. Unfortunately many people have found out the hard way that what is appropriate for football does not often transfer well to other sports. It is very easy to see that influence even today, because the term *strength and conditioning* evokes an image of training two separate qualities. It sends the wrong message. As you will see in the coming chapters, strength and conditioning are part of a much bigger picture. That big picture is developing complete athletes to be at their physical best and stay injury free in their chosen sports. A broader, more descriptive term that evokes the goal is *athletic development*. The goal is to train all the components of athleticism to the degree required by the sport that the athlete participates in. The athletic development coach is part of a performance team. A well-qualified athletic development coach usually makes a good leader of a performance team because that coach is well grounded in the big picture. The very nature of the job demands that the coach be the consummate generalist.

Athletic development coaches should be granted the same professional courtesy and respect as the sport coaches, but that respect must be earned. The only way it can be earned is if all people involved work to more clearly define their roles. It demands getting out of the weight room and broadening your horizons to incorporate training of all athletic qualities. The evolution of the role of the athletic trainer (ATC) should serve as a good model. Certified athletic trainers have certainly evolved into much more valued and prestigious figures than they were 40 years ago. They have done that by professionalizing and defining their field. Athletic development coaches must do the same. Athletic development coaches must develop a skill set consisting of a precise blend of what to coach and how to coach. All the technical knowledge in the world is for naught if the information cannot be imparted to athletes in a format and style that they can use. It is what you do with what you know. You need to have a clear distinction between coaching and personal training. Personal training is about appearance and pleasing the client. Athletic development coaching is about structure, long-term commitment, and training for performance.

Athletic development is the process of evaluating and training all the components of athleticism according to the demands of the sports and the qualities of the individual athlete. It is based on the understanding that athleticism is the ability to perform athletic movements (run, jump, and throw) at optimal speed with precision, style, and grace.

As an athletic development coach, you are a part of the whole development and training process. You are support staff. Keep things in balance. Do not claim credit for wins unless you are willing to accept blame for losses. Stay in the background; focus on the job of making the athletes better. The best self-promotion is a job well done.

Athletic development coaches should be evaluated based on their ability to train, improve, and refine the qualities of athleticism. Unfortunately, because the role of strength and conditioning coaches has been so closely tied to football, the strength coaches' evaluation is often tied to wins and losses. This is unfortunate. There are standards of professional behavior that must be upheld regardless of the field of coaching. Evaluation will become much more objective when the field is clearly defined.

The guru mentality has hindered the definition of the field. Certainly the growth of the Internet has contributed to this. To be an expert on the Internet, all you need to do is get a Web page and declare that you are an expert. Despite what these experts proclaim, there are no secret methods or hidden formulas. The information is out there and it should be shared, but it is up to each athletic development coach to take the information and formulate it into a system that applies to each particular situation. When you are looking for information, look for substance, not style. Look beyond the marketing and hype. Just because someone trained an athlete who was voted most valuable player or an all-star player does not mean that the coach knows everything. There is no substitute for experience; in fact, it is a great teacher, if you are willing to learn the lessons. Guiding someone from the beginning stages to stardom is the measure of substance. Dr. Joe Vigil worked with Deena Kastor for *eight* years to guide her to her marathon medal in Athens. Eight years and 40,000 miles of running are the measure of a great coach. When Dr. Vigil speaks, you know it is about substance, not style.

Constant evaluation should lead to change in order to improve. Sometimes change is very uncomfortable, but it is a constant in life and in coaching. Gandhi said, "You must be the change you wish to see in the world." That certainly is a challenge, but to be a great coach it is necessary. The following seven steps in the process will enable you to understand and manage change in your life and in your career:

Level 1: Effectiveness—doing the right thing

Level 2: Efficiency—doing things right

Level 3: Improving—doing the right things better

Level 4: Cutting—doing away with unessential things

Level 5: Copying—doing things well that other successful people are doing

Level 6: Different—doing things no one else is doing

Level 7: Impossible—doing things that can't be done

It is always better to manage change rather than have it manage you. Ben Franklin summed it up quite well: "When you are finished changing, you are finished." Remember that coaches are change agents; they are constantly working to change people to perform to optimal levels.

Remember the movement constants and the rules of training. Evaluate everything with those in mind and you will get to the destination on the functional path with a minimum of interference. Jerry Garcia said it best: "You do not merely want to be considered the best of the best. You want to be considered the only ones who do what you do." That is the challenge.

SUMMARY

The first step on the functional path is establishing a philosophy of coaching. It is the cornerstone on which a successful training program is built. This is your (and subsequently the athletes') guiding light. The philosophy should be evident in everything you do. Taking the time to formulate a philosophy may be one of the most important things that you can do to provide a steady direction for your athletes. Within this philosophy, you must bear in mind that the field of athletic development is evolving constantly. This is a reflection of the relative infancy of the field and the explosion of knowledge about training. This presents both a challenge and an opportunity. It will be a challenge to maintain a steady course and keep high professional standards. It is also an opportunity to innovate and to travel uncharted waters.

Factors Affecting
Athletic Movement

Effective movement, especially high-level athletic performance, is the result of the interplay of the three movement constants: the body, gravity, and the ground. Understanding each of the movement constants independently is one thing, but the real key is to understand how they interact. The enhancement of the interaction of the movement constants will move you farther down the functional path so that you can design the most effective training program for the athlete. This is both the art and science of training. To design and implement the most effective training program, never lose sight of the interaction of the three constants.

To further your understanding of movement on the functional path, you need to understand the movement constants and their interrelationships. The interaction of the three constants produces efficient athletic movement, so you must factor them into every training program.

MOVEMENT AND THE BODY

The first movement constant is the body. The body is a complex system designed to produce movements on demand for the required activity. The construction of the body reveals that there is a master design. There are various lever systems in which the body has a mechanical advantage in certain tasks and disadvantages in others. In many ways the body is a work in progress; it is highly adaptable to a variety of conditions and stresses.

You must understand the structure of the body in order to train the body for high-level performance. For example, look at the muscles of the thigh, the hamstrings, and the quadriceps. The quads, because of their high pennation angles, large cross-sectional area, and short fibers, are best used to produce large forces. The hamstrings (see figure 2.1), because of their longer fibers and smaller cross-sectional area, are designed to move in a large range of motions at speed (Lieber 2002). These relatively simple considerations of muscle architecture have huge implications in the selection of exercises to strengthen these muscles to work together to produce efficient movement.

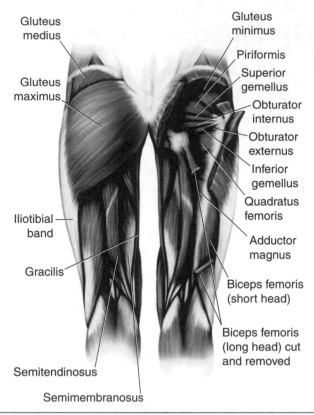

Figure 2.1 Posterior view of upper-leg muscles. The all-important hamstring muscles are very important in performance enhancement and injury prevention because of their structure and function in the body.

Connectivity of the Body Systems

There is a synergy between systems of the body. The neural, muscular, cardiovascular, and endocrinological (hormonal) systems all work simultaneously, not independently, to help the body maintain a state of homeostasis. Oschman (2003, p. 57) has proposed that "there must be a high-speed communication system in living systems that is not the nervous system; instead it is a body-wide energetic communication that includes the nervous, circulatory, and immune systems, and it also includes all of the other systems of the body. This system of systems has come to be called the living matrix." The communication system between all systems of the body is connective tissue, most specifically fascia. "The connective tissue forms a continuously interconnected system throughout the living body. All movements, of the body as a whole and of its smallest parts, are created by tensions carried through the connective tissue fabric" (Oschman 2003, p. 61). Often aches and pains from training are diagnosed as tendinitis or joint problems, but actually they are caused by fascial restrictions resulting from improper patterns of movement.

To be most effective, the emphasis in training must be on the interaction of all the systems of the body. Unfortunately, the textbook approach reinforces the segmentation of the systems. This approach to each system separately is mentally convenient, but it is a concept to avoid when training the body for optimal performance.

The fascial system and the central nervous system (CNS), the command and control system of the body, work closely together to transfer the neural impulses to trigger movement. It is highly plastic and programmable. Therefore, it is imperative to be aware of the input. Each activity is subjected to further refinements and adjustments by feedback from the body's proprioceptors. This process ensures optimal neuromuscular control and efficiency of function. If the system is fed faulty motor programs or the nervous system is confused with conflicting input, then output will be faulty. Each activity can be further refined and modified by sensory feedback from the body's proprioceptors. Work with stroke patients has shown that the circuitry of the brain can be "rewired" in as little as three weeks to enable stroke patients to regain function of a limb. When training athletes, I have found it helpful to think of that fact. They require that much patience and care to help them reach their potential. Their circuits are always open, and they can be rewired. This entire process of providing effective input ensures optimal neuromuscular control and efficiency of function.

Planes of Motion

The actual output is muscle function, which results in movement. This is perhaps the biggest paradigm shift caused by the increased awareness of functional training. The thinking must shift away from isolated muscles to patterns of movement and how the muscles actually function within those patterns. Because anatomy and clinical muscle function are taught from a position of mental convenience and emphasize the concentric function of an isolated area, this results in some confusion. For example, in textbook anatomy, the hamstrings' main function is defined as a flexor of the knee. In actual movement, the hamstrings help with flexion of the knee, but that is not their primary job. Their primary job is to work eccentrically to decelerate the lower leg and extend the hip. The function changes with the orientation of the body to gravity and the ground. Movement does not occur only in the sagittal plane. According to Enoka (1994), the function of a muscle depends critically on the context in which it is activated. As part of one movement, a muscle can perform a certain way; in another movement it is capable of doing the exact opposite. Movement is complex, requiring the interaction of multiple muscle systems in all three planes of motion. It occurs in reaction to gravity, ground reaction forces (GRF), and momentum.

Movement is a complex event that involves synergists, stabilizers, neutralizers, and antagonists all working together to produce efficient movement in all three planes of motion. The cornerstone of functional training and rehabilitation is to train movements, not muscles. The muscles are slaves of the brain. The brain does not recognize isolated muscles; it recognizes patterns of movement in response to sensory input from the environment. Training isolated movements (individual muscles) has the potential to create tremendous neural confusion. This is something to avoid at all costs. It may be more convenient to train an individual muscle, but it complicates the process of getting that muscle to work as part of an integrated whole.

The three cardinal planes of movements are sagittal, frontal, and transverse (see figure 2.2). The sagittal plane divides the body into right and left sides. In many respects it is the dominant plane of movement because gait (walking) occurs in the sagittal plane, and gait is the root of all movement. I call it the plane of convenience. It is the plane in which most action pictures are taken. Most exercise progressions begin in the sagittal plane because of the familiarity of movement in this plane. In program design and exercise selection, it is important not to fixate on the sagittal plane.

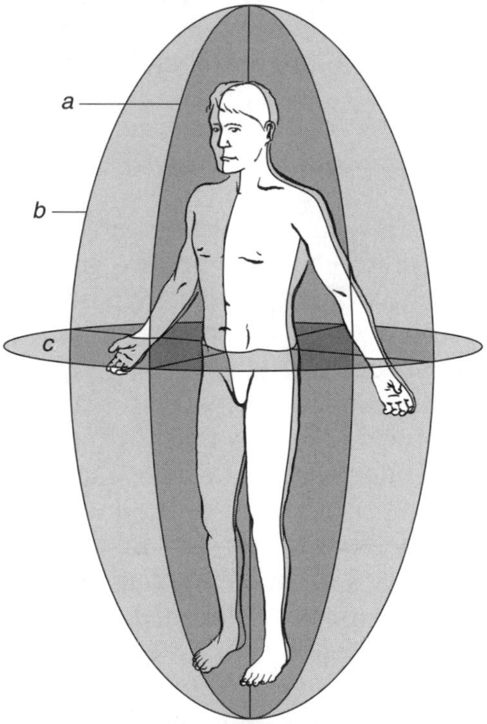

The frontal plane divides the front and back of the body. It involves sideways movement. The transverse plane divides the top and bottom of the body. Rotational movement occurs in this plane. It is probably the most misunderstood and most important of the three planes of motion. Unfortunately, rotational movement is portrayed as dangerous. Nothing could be further from reality. Rotation and the ability to control rotational forces are essential to efficient injury-free movement. From a training and performance standpoint, if one plane is more important than the others, then the transverse plane is most important because it involves rotation and is the plane in which the most common injuries occur: ankle sprains, ACL tears, hamstring pulls. The body

Figure 2.2 The three planes of movement: (a) the sagittal plane, (b) the frontal plane, and (c) the transverse plane. The three planes of movement allow us to more accurately describe movement, which in turn helps us to more accurately select appropriate functional exercises.

does a tremendous amount of work in this plane to decelerate external forces. Therefore a significant portion of strength training and core work is focused on the transverse plane.

Essentially movement is triplanar (that is, involving the three planes), usually in diagonal rotational patterns. According to Logan and McKinney (1970, p. 158), "there also appears to be some neurologic bases for diagonal movement patterns. One reflex adds some credibility to the diagonal movement pattern, the crossed extensor reflex. Simply stated, this reflex is a combination of the flexion reflex in one limb and the extensor reflex occurring simultaneously in the opposite limb. This crossed extensor reflex is responsible for an 'automatic relationship' in diagonal type movements." Movement occurs in all three planes at the same time. This is the argument against building a strength training program with the use of machines. Most machines allow movement in only one plane, most often the sagittal plane. Triplanar movement also requires a paradigm shift because it is more difficult to visualize and articulate. It is certainly simpler and more convenient to look at movement in one plane with one muscle working, but that is not how it works in real life.

As a coach, I think of the feedback from the athlete when she "gets it." I may have worked on a particular aspect of movement for a period when the athlete "gets it." The comment is "That felt easy" or "I wasn't even trying." The athlete "getting it" is evidence of the integration, the feeling for the whole, the flow that is produced by efficient triplanar movement. I have seldom had an athlete get it by working on an isolated segment. The result was very uncoordinated movement, not a flow.

Movement Terminology

Along with shifting thinking regarding muscle function, it would be beneficial to revisit some basic terminology in regard to movement. Traditionally terms such as *prime mover* and *antagonist* have been used. But these terms can limit us and lock us into the same pattern of looking at muscles rather than movements. In their classic text *Kinesiology*, last published in 1970, Logan and McKinney proposed the use of terminology that fits with our contemporary understanding of muscle function. Their logic in proposing a shift in terminology is as on target today as when they first articulated it: The terms *agonist, antagonist, synergist*, and *fixator* are used to describe muscle action. But these terms do not describe muscle actions because they have been used in a context that has not considered the effects of gravity as well as other external forces acting on and within the body.

Terminology is important because it facilitates communication. Words create images and images create action. Shifting to the terminology provided by Logan and McKinney (1970) will help to further an understanding of functional movement:

- **Muscle most involved (MMI)** is the muscle that overcomes resistance and moves a joint through a specified plane of motion.
- **Contralateral muscle** works with the muscle most involved (MMI).
- **Guiding muscle** helps rule out and control undesired action.
- **Stabilizing muscle** holds a joint or a body part to enable other body parts or joints to move efficiently.

A better understanding of muscle function will allow training to be more focused, logical, and exact and will help you do a better job of selecting equipment. It will also enable the design of equipment that is more functional. The focus shifts from "feel the burn" and "no pain, no gain" to an understanding and feeling of flow and rhythm in the movements.

MOVEMENT AND GRAVITY

The second movement constant is gravity. All work and play occur in a gravitationally enriched environment. Movement is gravity driven. Movement is a delicate balance yielding to gravity or being able to overcome it.

Sport performance involves learning how to cheat gravity. Occasionally humans beat gravity for an instant, but gravity is relentless. A good portion of the musculature of the body functions in daily activities as "antigravity" muscles to keep the body upright. Aging is an example of gravity winning. If you observe people through their life span, they get shorter and begin to stoop over as time goes on. But small interventions of strength training for people in their 70s and 80s have dramatic effects on posture and bone structure. Essentially strength training in the older population cheats gravity to help overcome the effects of aging.

Performance Paradigm

I use the performance paradigm as a tool to illustrate the interrelationship of the components of movement and as a guide in determining how to train all components. The performance paradigm is a model to illustrate how gravity loads the system to initiate movement (see figure 2.3). The structure of the body is designed to resist the constant pull of gravity toward the center of the earth. Essentially all movement is interplay between force reduction and force production. The quality of the movement is regulated by the proprioceptive system. The paradigm also serves as a guide in evaluating movement from a different context (see the table in figure 2.3). It emphasizes the timing and sequence of all three components of the paradigm. The interplay between force reduction, force production, and proprioception will produce the highest quality of movement.

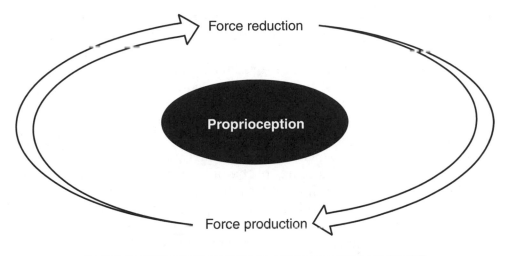

Force production	Force reduction
Against gravity	With gravity
Concentric	Eccentric
Acceleration	Deceleration
Acting	Reacting
Overcoming	Accommodating
Extending	Bending
Unloading	Loading
Proprioception	
Joint position awareness—occurs at the subcortical level	

Figure 2.3 The performance paradigm schematically represents the interplay of force reduction, force production, and proprioception.

We begin movement by loading the muscles—this is the force-reduction phase. A stretched muscle can exert more force. Muscles function as shock-absorbing structures and springs when they absorb mechanical work while eccentrically lengthening. The forces from these eccentric muscle contractions produce negative work (LaStayo et al. 2003). Basically this is the eccentric loading phase. This may be the most important component of the performance paradigm but probably the most overlooked as well as the most misunderstood. The most notable reason is that it is not very measurable. Because it is difficult to quantify, we have tended to emphasize the more measurable component, force production. Most injuries occur during the force-reduction phase. It is during this phase that gravity has its greatest impact; it is literally trying to slam the body into the ground. The shock-absorbing and springlike capabilities afford unlimited opportunities to explore this component for performance enhancement and rehabilitation.

Once force has been reduced, the result is force production. Force production is easy to see and easy to measure. Consequently it gets an inordinate amount of attention in the training process. We see it because it is the outcome of the eccentric loading in the force-reduction phase. It is how high or far we jump and how much we lift. It is one component of the performance paradigm that is highly dependent on the other phases.

Proprioception is in the center of the performance paradigm because it is the unifying element that enables force production and force reduction to be controlled and guided. Proprioception is the awareness of joint position and force derived from the sensory receptors in the joints, ligaments, muscles, and tendons. From a coaching perspective, proprioception is the component that gives the quality to the movement; it determines how the muscle will respond. As Logan and McKinney (1970, p. 62) point out, "The quality of movement, in part, is dependent upon neurologic information fed back from proprioceptors within muscles and joints to the higher brain centers. The information returning to the central nervous system from the periphery includes 'data' concerning tension of muscle fibers, joint angles, and position of the body being moved." It is the feedback mechanism that positions the limbs to be able to achieve optimal efficiency. Any change in muscle length, tension, joint position, or motion is closely monitored by the receptor systems of the body. Any changes that are monitored are then sent to the spinal cord, the brain stem, and the cortex to fine-tune muscle function to improve precision, accuracy, and strength of movement. Proprioception is the component of movement that has been all but ignored in most traditional training programs until recently. It is highly trainable, especially if it is incorporated as part of a whole program. We go into detail on how to accomplish this in subsequent chapters.

Antigravity Muscles

When the body is not moving, it may appear static, but in actuality the body is in constant motion as it reacts to the force of gravity. One of the main functions of the muscles is to maintain an upright position. Maintenance of this position requires significant integrated activity of the large muscle groups of the body. Logan and McKinney (1970) have termed the muscles that are most active in resisting the force of gravity the *antigravity muscles*. The antigravity muscles make possible the maintenance of body postures in sport, exercise, and dance. The following four muscle groups are the primary antigravity muscle groups: the gastrocnemius and soleus groups, the quadriceps group, and the erector spinae group. When the body is upright, as is the case in many sport activities, the antigravity muscle groups work in conjunction with other muscle groups to maintain an upright posture. This concept has broad implications in all components of training, which are detailed in subsequent chapters.

MOVEMENT AND THE GROUND

The third movement constant is the ground. The ground is where we live, work, and play. A goal of training is to learn to use the ground to our best advantage. The role of the ground in movement is something martial arts practitioners have understood for thousands of years. Human movement in relation to the ground has the following qualities:

Rooted in the feet

Powered by the core

Reflected by the arms

Manifested in the hands

Movement begins at the ground. Everything is expressed from the ground upward; consequently, all movement is a reflection of the quality of being rooted. The natural analogy of the tree is particularly appropriate. The size and strength of the trunk are not ultimately what determine the strength of the tree; it is the root structure. As you proceed down the functional path to build the complete athlete, keep this analogy in mind. The way that

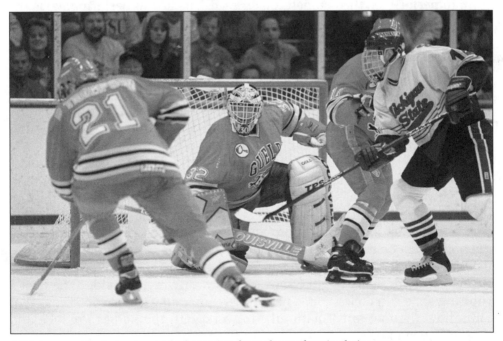

Athletes must train to use ground reaction from the surface in their sport.

force is imparted into the ground and the subsequent ground reaction go a long way to determine the quality of the athlete's performance. The ability to use the ground effectively plays a significant role in injury prevention and rehabilitation.

In relation to the ground, the terms *open chain* and *closed chain* have gained popularity both in coaching and in scientific literature. The conventional definitions of *open chain* as the distal segment of a limb free in space and *closed chain* as the distal segment fixed on the ground lead us to believe that each is a discrete and separate event. In fact, movement is ultimately the timing of the opening and closing of the chain. Gait is a great example of this. The stance leg is in contact (briefly) with the ground; therefore gait is closed-chain movement. Conversely, the swing leg is free; therefore it is open. In reality it is impossible to separate the two. Efficient gait is the interaction and timing of the opening and closing of the chain. Because the terms are somewhat artificial, they are not used in this text unless they can enhance a concept or a training method.

The gait cycle is the cornerstone of function that enables the human body to use the ground effectively. There are few activities in sport and life where people do activities off of two feet. Most activities are reciprocal, beginning off one foot and moving to the other foot, as in gait. Therefore, as a fundamental movement, gait is the basis of most of the exercise patterns.

Obviously in enhancement of sport performance, the athlete must be able to perform on a variety of surfaces. Surfaces occur on a continuum from hard to soft and even to uneven. To effectively perform, the athlete must train to perform on the competition surface. The key to performance is the ability to import force into the ground, whatever surface, and in turn derive appropriate useable ground reaction. The ability to control and use ground reaction force has implications in regard to movement mechanics, strength training, injury prevention, and rehabilitation. To design and implement effective training and rehabilitation programs, you need to understand how to use and control ground reaction force. It is also important to understand the effects of repetitive activities where ground reaction force is lower but the cumulative stress effect can be quite high.

One of the typical solutions in controlling and dissipating ground reaction force has been to make the shoe more controlling and shock absorbent. This has actually created more problems than it has solved. It is helpful to think of the shoe as the interface between the foot and ground. The shoe cannot make up for what the body is incapable of doing. The structures of the body must be trained to reduce the force over as many joints as possible using the elastic properties of the muscles, ligaments, and tendons. Coleman Horn, former designer of Nike shoes, put it best when he said, "The best a running shoe can do for you is not hinder your gait." Choose footwear that will allow the foot to act naturally, to work with the body to reduce and then produce force.

SUMMARY

The understanding of the movement constants and their interplay and relationship is a huge step toward designing functional training programs. The constants are the basics, in essence the alphabet of training. It is easy to get caught up in training methods and exercises and lose sight of the constants. If you do lose sight of the constants, then the training programs will not be effective. The foundation for effectively applying the concept of the movement constants to the implementation of actual training is the performance paradigm. This paradigm is a simple representation of the interplay of forces acting on the body. Use this paradigm to check your programs so that there is a balance between force production and force reduction properly guided by proprioception.

Sport-Specific Demands Analysis

Now that you have a basic understanding of muscle function and a handle on the movement constants, you can explore what you need to do to design an effective training program for any sport. You must have an understanding of the sport you are conditioning for. A failure to completely evaluate sport demands manifests itself later as performance errors, injuries, or overtraining. Do not make assumptions about sports and positions or events within a respective sport.

Digital video and computer analyses have significantly advanced the field of notational analysis. We now have exact information on movement in games. However, much of the effort has been directed toward analysis of techniques, tactics, and strategies. Not much analysis has been directed toward identifying conditioning components. Regardless, the information is invaluable from the perspective of the conditioning coach. It is possible to derive information about velocities at various times in the game, patterns of movement, frequency of certain actions, and comparison of actions at various points in the game to determine fatigue. Most coaches do not have these sophisticated tools available to them. It's great if you have them available, but you can get the job done with simple tools coupled with a systematic approach to the analysis.

SYSTEMATIC SPORT ANALYSIS MODEL

You can achieve a systematic approach to sport analysis at any level by following a simple four-step process. The four steps are analyze the demands of the sport, understand the position or event in the sport, analyze the qualities of the athlete, and understand the common injuries in the sport. This comprehensive model directs everything in a training program and gives you the ability to work with a variety of sports. You do not need to be an expert in the sport; you just need to be able to objectively work through all four steps to design a specific conditioning program to fit the particular sport.

1. Analyze the Demands of the Sport

What type of sport is it? What are the patterns of movement? What are the rules? This information has a significant impact on the sport. For example, the length of quarters, shot clock, and width of the lane all have a significant impact on basketball. Therefore, preparing a team at the high school level can be significantly different from preparing a team at the professional level. The difference is more than the level of ability and talent.

Tactics have a significant effect on sport demands. In American football an option offense has very different demands than a passing offense. This can even be a factor in an individual sport such as tennis, in which one player can be a serve-and-volley player and another a baseline player. Both players are playing on the same dimensions of the court, but they are playing vastly different games.

You will need to avoid assumptions and base training on a thorough demands analysis. The eye opener for me came in 1987 when I was assistant conditioning coach for the Chicago Bulls. I did an isolated video analysis of our top six players in games. The results were shocking. I had been fooled into believing the hype of NBA basketball as show-time, high-paced action played above the rim. But the opposite was true. Most of the game was played below the rim. Only one player ran the length of the floor, the power forward who took the ball out of bounds. The point guards basically moved from the top of the key to the top of the key. The game was played at a jogging pace. The conditioning implications were obvious. We were doing entirely too much aerobic work. We needed to shift the emphasis to more power activities and power endurance. The lesson I learned is to take the time to gain an in-depth understanding of the game before designing a training program.

Start by classifying the sport into categories. Most sports fall into categories that share common characteristics. Some sports overlap classifications; with those sports it is best to assign a classification system based on experience with the sport and the athletes you are working with. The following are the four broad categories of sports:

- **Sprint sport.** These sports require all-out maximum effort. The goal is to achieve as fast a time as possible for the prescribed distance. The ability to recover or quickly repeat the effort is not a factor. The sprint events in track are examples of sprint sports.

- **Intermittent-sprint sport.** These sports require a series of maximum efforts with time for relatively full recovery between efforts. American football, rugby, ice hockey, and volleyball are examples.

- **Transition-game sport.** These sports require a series of efforts of varied intensity that occur in random patterns. Recovery between efforts varies from almost nonexistent to close to complete. Soccer, field hockey, and lacrosse are examples.

- **Endurance sport.** These sports are characterized by continual submaximal effort with the goal to finish in the shortest time possible for a certain distance. This is subdivided by duration into short term (1 to 20 minutes), medium term (20 to 60 minutes), and long term (more than 60 minutes).

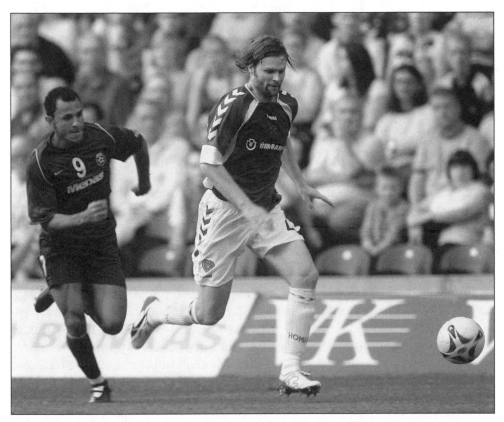

A transition-game sport like soccer requires conditioning that addresses the game's varied intensity and recovery times.

© Empics

Sports that fall into this classification are the typical endurance sports such as the marathon and triathlon.

Some sports fall in between categories because they have characteristics of intermittent-sprint and transition-game sports. Tennis and basketball are examples of this. In cases like this you need to consider how the game is played by the team or player that you are working with and then condition accordingly. Remember that these are just guidelines, not hard-and-fast rules.

There are some additional factors that you must take into consideration when considering sport demands. Differentiating between noncontact, contact, collision, and impact is an important factor for determining training emphasis. Examples of a contact sport are basketball and soccer. Contact is considered incidental but still must be considered as a training factor. Sports such as American football, ice hockey, and rugby are collision sports because physically stopping the opponent is essential to success in the game. That dictates an emphasis in strength training to develop bulk for protection, which has profound implications on the type and frequency of strength training as well as the recovery protocols. I classify impact sports as those activities in which landing forces are very high or lower forces are repeated for a prolonged period. As an example of the latter, the average distance runner takes approximately 3,000 foot strikes per mile. Running requires each leg to bear the weight of the entire body because both feet never touch the ground at the same time. The force of landing is approximately three times the body weight. That means a 150-pound (68 kg) runner is placing 450 pounds (204 kg) of force on each leg in every stride. Gymnastics and triple jump are examples of high-impact forces for very short duration. In either scenario, impact forces will dictate the type of remedial injury prevention component.

2. Understand the Position or Event in the Sport

The next step in the systematic sport analysis model is to understand the position or the event in the sport. In American football, there are 22 players on the field. Each of the positions has different demands. Some positions are quite similar and others are quite different. Because they are all playing the same game, there should be some commonality in their training, but there should also be some distinct differences. The demands on a quarterback are significantly different than the demands on a defensive tackle. Look closely at the pattern of movement, speed requirements, strength requirements, and specific endurance requirements. In basketball the demands for a post player are different than for a perimeter player. In soccer the forward has very different conditioning needs than the defender based on the movement demands of their respective positions.

A thorough analysis of sport demands should incorporate an analysis of the demands of the various positions and events. This has been the biggest change in my approach to conditioning. Careful consideration of the differing demands of various positions in a specific sport has had a profound effect on how I prepare the athletes. The results have been much more consistent, reproducible, and on target. I have also noticed a significant motivational benefit: The athletes definitely relate to what they are doing because they can see the direct application to their performance.

3. Analyze the Qualities of the Athlete

The third step is to consider the qualities that each athlete brings to the sport. Consider the training age. Training age is how long the athlete has been in formal training for the sport. The level of development in the sport has significant impact. Is the athlete a novice or a highly advanced performer? Also consider the physical qualities. How fast, how strong, how powerful, how fit is the athlete? What is the person's skill level? All of this can be evaluated through game analysis and actual testing of the physical capacities (see chapter 4). This is a great deal of work, but it is definitely worth the effort. Careful consideration of each individual's qualities is probably the biggest factor that will ensure success of a conditioning program.

4. Understand the Common Injuries in the Sport

Assess the pattern of injuries or the common injuries that occur in the sport. This is an important measure in keeping the athlete healthy. Understanding this enables you to place an effective injury-prevention component in the overall plan. For example, we know that baseball pitching puts inordinate stress on the shoulder and elbow. The training program must reflect this. Remember that high-level athletic fitness is a fine edge. I heard a speaker at a sports medicine symposium say that a healthy athlete is an oxymoron. To excel to elite levels, the athlete must push the limits at various times in training. This elevates the risk and makes it imperative to have a well-thought-out plan with variation in loading that enables the athlete to tolerate the training. Nevertheless, if you understand the common injuries and patterns in a sport, then you can go a long way in preventing them. Also, by better understanding injury patterns and stresses, you will be better able to design effective rehabilitation programs if the athlete does get injured.

SPORT DEMANDS ANALYSIS

A method that I use to analyze the overall demands of team sports is the focal point approach. Looking for a focal point in a sport has helped me to focus on the key movements and key positions and then condition accordingly. Certain focal points are the determining factors for success in the respective sports. For example, in baseball the catcher is the focal point of the game. If you draw concentric circles out from the catcher with the catcher and pitcher in the first circle; the first baseman, third baseman, and middle infielders in the second circle; and the outfielders in the last circle, it will define movement patterns. In soccer the focal point is often the central midfielders. In volleyball it is the setter. In football it is the center and quarterback. Each subsequent concentric circle out from the focal point will have distinct demands and movement patterns. Find the focal point in the sport you are working with and design the training around this focal point.

To be more precise in assessing the demands of the sport in order to direct training, I have designed an instrument called the sport demands analysis (SDA), which is displayed in figure 3.1. This is a tool that helps me focus on the need to do activities that will make the athletes better in that sport. I have used this in situations where I have had only a peripheral familiarity with a sport because it helped me focus on essential components of the sport.

Figure 3.1

SPORT DEMANDS ANALYSIS

Physical Demands
(1 = low, 10 = high)

Aerobic endurance	1	2	3	4	5	6	7	8	9	10
Speed	1	2	3	4	5	6	7	8	9	10
Agility	1	2	3	4	5	6	7	8	9	10
Strength	1	2	3	4	5	6	7	8	9	10
Power	1	2	3	4	5	6	7	8	9	10
Skill	1	2	3	4	5	6	7	8	9	10

Sport Characteristics

☐ Team   ☐ Individual   ☐ Aquatic

☐ Artistic   ☐ Combative   ☐ Collision

☐ Contact   ☐ Impact   ☐ Equipment dominant

Length of Competition

Time of actual competition (actual activity in the game)

_____

_____

_____

_____

Work-to-rest ratio (in the competition)

_____

_____

_____

_____

Distribution of intensity of effort (How frequently is all-out effort required?)

1	2	3	4	5	6	7	8	9	10

Infrequent   Frequent
maximal effort   maximal effort

From V. Gambetta, 2007, *Athletic development: The art & science of functional sports conditioning*, (Champaign, IL: Human Kinetics).

Temporal Classification

☐ Set time frame   ☐ Open time frame

_____

_____

_____

_____

The Competitive Season

☐ Length of season   ☐ Multiple seasons
☐ Number of competitions   ☐ Competition frequency
☐ Championship format

_____

_____

_____

_____

From V. Gambetta, 2007, _Athletic development: The art & science of functional sports conditioning_, (Champaign, IL: Human Kinetics).

Each sport has different characteristics in different proportions. Use the SDA to rate the sport as you see it and to focus on the key actions that take place in the game. It is an instrument that is easily adaptable to many situations. Each coach can personalize it to his or her respective situation. The SDA should provide you with direction and trends; it is not meant to be absolute. Keep observing, and modify it as needed. Using the SDA periodically can also serve as a good self-scouting tool in spotting any trends in training that could cause problems later on.

The emphasis is on the overall pattern of play, not just what is happening at the ball. Focusing on just the ball and what happens around the ball is too narrow. That is not where all the action occurs. You need to see how action develops—how the player _got to_ the ball is also important. Today much of our conditioning is biased by the "highlight play syndrome." We see clips of spectacular plays daily on TV, when in reality those plays occur infrequently, sometimes only once a season. Resist this influence when designing a conditioning program. The program must condition athletes for what happens on a consistent basis.

Beware of the trickle-down effect, where there is a natural tendency to look at a sport performed at the highest level and then adapt it to the lower developmental levels of the sport. The level of play, length of periods of play, time clock, and rules can significantly change a game. This in turn affects the emphasis on conditioning. For example, there is a big difference between basketball played under international rules and basketball played under NBA rules, and in turn it has significant conditioning implications, not to mention tactical and strategic implications.

Sometimes proficiency can be a liability rather than an asset. I have heard this statement many times: "That's the way I played the game." My retort is, "That's how you *thought* you played the game." Be objective in analysis, not biased by your ability or lack of ability to play the game. I know how I trained for the decathlon, which is not how I trained my athletes. They were world class, at a much higher level than I ever was, and that indicated that their training needs were quite different from mine. Certainly experience with the sport is helpful if that experience is used as a reference point.

APPLICATION OF SPORT ANALYSIS

Performance analysis ensures a relatively easy and accurate recall of performance. Instead of relying on memory, which tends to be inaccurate, it provides objective markers. Analysis offers the ability to assess quality of play to determine position on the team or performance ranking outside the win–loss column. Good analysis will track players' movement so that you can analyze patterns and style of play, which you can use to design more specific training programs for an individual or team.

Let's look closely at the sport of basketball and work through an evaluation of notational analysis and biomechanics data to gain some insights to design an effective conditioning and injury-prevention program. The following data were derived from analysis of a game in the Australian National Basketball League (McInnes et al. 1995). The rules dictate that the game consists of four 12-minute quarters, 2-minute breaks between quarters, and a 15-minute halftime. The following movements occurred during the game. The total duration of each activity during the course of the game is as follows:

Walking or standing: 4 minutes

Jogging: 4 minutes

Running: 4 minutes

Sprinting: 3 minutes

Shuffling at low to medium intensity: 9 minutes

Shuffling at high intensity: 2 minutes

Jumping: 41 seconds

While the ball was in play, there was a change in movement category every two seconds. This resulted in more than 1,000 different movements during a game. This is a very significant fact, because it indicated the high-intensity quick changes in movements demanded by the game. This study did not break down the analysis by position, but it should be pointed out that that there will be some differences between the data for a perimeter player and a post player. The following data provide even more specific information to direct conditioning:

Of the total court time, 28 percent was spent in strenuous exertion.

Intense activity occured in bursts of 13 to 14 seconds at a time.

There were 105 high-intensity efforts per game.

There was an intense effort every 21 seconds.

This provides the necessary information to design the conditioning approach in terms of frequency and intensity of effort. From this we can design workouts with work-to-rest ratios that reflect the demands of the game. We can determine volume of work based on number of intense efforts that occur in the game. This is an area that must be emphasized in order to achieve optimal levels of game fitness. Arbitrary volumes are not exact; game analysis data can provide exact ranges in terms of volume of work.

The following data provide information on direction of movement that will help you to design a more specific multidimensional speed and agility program:

Side-to-side movements made up 31 percent of the game.

Two-thirds of these movements were intense.

Individual shuffle movements were 1 to 4 seconds in duration.

Sprints were 1 to 5 seconds in duration.

This information indicates that the movements are of very high intensity. The training should reflect this. If this were all the information available, it would certainly be enough to design a specific basketball conditioning program. Some additional research statistics on NBA players give even better insight into the game in terms of forces (McClay et al. 1994a and 1994b). These studies were driven by the need to identify the causes of stress fractures. They are a combination of game analysis and biomechanical lab tests. Nonetheless, the information derived is invaluable in terms of designing and implementing a specific strength and plyometric training program.

To assess the intensity of jumping, the jumps were classified as low, medium, or high intensity. A low-intensity jump usually occurred at a shot or an unchallenged rebound. A medium-intensity jump encompassed most rebounds, defending jump shots, and a jump shot. A high-intensity jump occurred in a maximal or near-maximal effort, as would occur with a dunk blocked shot or a challenged jump shot. During a game, 30 percent of the jumps were low intensity, 45 percent were medium intensity, and 25 percent were high intensity. The average number of jumps per game was 70. The range of jumps for different positions was 55 for guards, 83 for centers, and 72 for forwards.

The conclusion that I derived from these data was that the majority of jumps were of low and medium intensity. Therefore, the amount of plyometric work outside of practice and games, given the number of games and practices in a year, should be kept quite low. The kinetic data in table 3.1 are quite revealing about the actual forces in the various movements that occur in basketball.

In regard to injury, which was the focus of the studies, the following conclusion was derived: The forces, combined with 32 degrees of rearfoot supination and the large number of shuffling steps taken during a game, increase the stress on the lateral border of the foot, placing the fifth metatarsal at higher risk. Of all lower-extremity fractures in basketball, 52 percent are fractures of the fifth metatarsal (McClay et al. 1994a). These data tell me that I must focus on working the muscles as shock absorbers in order to attenuate the forces demanded in the various movements of the game.

The distance run in the course of a game seems to be a figure that attracts much attention, some of it unwarranted. In the course of a game it is not surprising that a typical NBA player runs 2.1 miles (about 3.4 km) at an average pace of 9 miles per hour (about 14.5 km/h), which is 6 minutes, 45 seconds per mile, or 4 minutes, 12 seconds per kilometer. These data are used to justify the amount of slow aerobic work that is prescribed. This ignores the key fact of the varied intensity of the movements. The fact that

Table 3.1   Ground Reaction Forces

Running
Vertical forces: 3 × body weight
Anterior and posterior forces: .5 × body weight
Mediolateral forces: .25 × body weight
Vertical forces
Starting: .8 × body weight
Lay-up landing: 8.9 × body weight
Stopping: 2.7 × body weight
Cutting: 3 × body weight
Anterior and posterior forces
Stopping: 1.3 × body weight
Mediolateral forces
Shuffling: 1.4 × body weight

Adapted, by permission, from I.S. McClay et al., 1994, "A profile of ground reaction forces in professional basketball," *Journal of Applied Biomechanics* 10(3): 221-236.

there are 1,000 shuffling movements during the game provides better information for conditioning the players to be better at the game and to prevent injury (McClay et al. 1994a).

How can we take these data and transfer them into a useable training program? First, look at the game as a series of intermittent, high-intensity, multidirectional movements. That will direct us immediately to high-intensity activities that involve varied movement patterns with variable work-to-rest ratios. The work will vary depending on the time of the training year and the state of fitness of the player. The immediate implication that we can derive from this analysis of basketball is that power is at a premium and that jumping of varied intensities and quick movements should be emphasized. We need to get away from the idea that the endurance base is built by long, slow, steady aerobic work. This type of work severely compromises explosiveness by preferentially recruiting slow-twitch fibers. Repetition of high-intensity work can raise aerobic capacity; therefore the training should be built around this type of work. Endurance for basketball or for other transition-game sports should be trained with general and game-specific (that is, imitation) drills in an intermittent pattern. A well-planned program can develop the endurance base necessary for enhancement of the aerobic fitness component without compromising explosive power.

SUMMARY

Good analysis of the sport will allow you to be more exact in training. It will allow you to be very specific and allow the appropriate adjustment of volumes and intensities in training to better reflect the game's demands. It is motivational for the athlete because the program can be personalized to each athlete's style and pattern of play. This is not to imply that all training should be limited to the specific movements of the game. There is a definite role for general preparation activities. Game analysis will bring objectivity to training, and bias will be eliminated.

If there is a secret to the whole process, it is making sure that you have as thorough an understanding of the game that you are preparing for as you possibly can. The tools that are available today to help you do this are easily accessible. This process will make the training more exact and specific to the sport and the athlete.

Options and Methods of Testing

Once you understand how the body moves and the demands on the body from various sports, you need to determine what physical qualities the athlete brings to the sport. Testing is used in identifying both strengths and weaknesses in speed, power, strength, and flexibility. This process enables you to personalize the program and make it specific to the sport and the athlete.

Testing is quantitative and objective. From testing you can derive hard numbers that you can use in a variety of ways. Evaluation, on the other hand, is qualitative and subjective; it indicates trends and ideas. The two combined provide the necessary information for devising the most precise training plan possible. Testing should assess the global motor qualities of the athlete and should reflect the demands of the sport. For example, the new hurdle flexibility tests presented later in this chapter give immediate feedback to the coach and athlete. From this feedback you can quickly devise a plan that should become a daily flexibility routine to address the deficiencies. There are several reasons for testing:

- It provides information and feedback on training progress. Where is the athlete relative to his or her goals?
- It will help you obtain information on specific components of an athlete's preparation. Testing will show whether the athlete is improving or regressing in a specific area.
- It can be used to predict future performance.
- It can indicate the athlete's readiness to return to play after an injury. If there are baseline data on the athlete, the athlete must reach a certain percentage of those baseline scores before returning to play.

Testing enables you to personalize the training program and set appropriate performance goals. Sometimes there is a tendency to take testing out of context and make it more than it is. It is essentially the highest training stress outside of actual competition. It must be recognized as such. Conversely, daily training is also testing. The results of daily training give a snapshot of the athlete's progress on a daily basis. Therefore, training equals testing, and testing equals training. Significantly more time is spent in training than in testing or competing, so remember to think of each training session as an opportunity to get feedback. Philosophically, test results should not be a factor in team selection. Team selection should be the result of performance in the competitive arena. There is no question that the physical and athletic qualities tested should contribute to actual sport performance, but it is still performance in the competitive arena that should be the deciding factor in team selection.

I differentiate evaluation from testing because evaluation is subjective. Evaluation is part of the daily process of training for both the coach and the athlete. Every workout should be carefully recorded with the subjective analysis of the workout. Were the goals of the workout achieved? If not, why weren't they achieved? Perhaps the most simple and effective means of monitoring training is for the athlete to keep a detailed training log. This is addressed in detail in chapter 14.

Each competition must be carefully analyzed and evaluated. It is imperative to look beyond the actual competition result to understand why the result occurred. Objective competition analysis will reveal patterns that result in good or bad competitive efforts. Competition analysis also should provide feedback on the preparation. Competition can verify that the plan is working or indicate the need for revision. The competition analysis should include the following:

- Time of day
- Weather conditions
- Field conditions, if applicable
- Warm-up
- Injuries (when and how they occurred)
- Subject's fatigue rating after the game or competition

Use all of this information to learn from each competition and make any necessary adjustments.

TEST SELECTION AND TIMING

Testing falls into two categories: criteria tests and progress checks. The criteria test is a battery of tests administered a maximum of three times in a yearly training cycle. Criteria tests are designed to assess the athlete's ability in regard to the global motor qualities (GMQ). Progress checks, on the other hand, are administered at various planned set points to assess training progress (see figure 4.1). The progress check is very specific. It is often designed to assess one specific motor quality; many times the progress check can be sport specific. Certainly progress checks will vary with the phase of the training year.

When you set out to select the tests and begin to define the testing protocols, don't be afraid to ask yourself the obvious question, "Why am I testing?" Are you testing because everyone else does, or do you have specific goals

Figure 4.1
SAMPLE PROGRESS CHECK TEST

Progress check test: High school hurdler or long jumper.

Phase of training: Start of special preparation phase.

Purpose of test: To evaluate explosive power following a phase of volume loading. Results were expected to be down, but all tests were at or near the athlete's best, which indicated that he adapted well to the loading. The next testing will be off a rubberized runway after an intensification cycle immediately before the beginning of a competition phase. We should see significant improvement on the tests. In fact, the results should approach the optimal numbers.

Conditions: 62 degrees Fahrenheit (16.7 Celsius), windy, light drizzle

Surface: Grass

Jump Test Results

Standing long jump
Best: 8 feet, 7 1/2 inches (2.63 meters)

Range: 7 inches (17.8 centimeters)

Rating: Good

Outstanding would be 10 feet (3.05 meters) or better

Standing triple jump
Best: 25 feet, 1 inch (7.65 meters)

Range: 1 foot, 11 inches (.58 meter)

Rating: Fair

Outstanding would be 30 feet (9.1 meters) plus

Five hops and jump (right and left)
Right—Best: 53 feet, 10 inches (16.41 meters)

Range: 2 feet, 10 inches (.86 meter)

Left—Best: 54 feet (16.46 meters)

Range: 3 feet, 6 inches (1.01 meters)

Difference: 2 inches (5 centimeters)

Rating: Outstanding

Anything under 18 inches (45.7 centimeters) difference right to left is outstanding

Five bounds and jump
Best: 50 feet (15.24 meters)

Range: 9 inches (22.86 centimeters)

Rating: Poor

Outstanding would be 58 feet (17.68 meters) or better

and objectives in mind? Just as with training, where it is possible to do too much, you can do too much in testing. I made that mistake with a group of decathletes I was coaching. I had a battery of progress checks consisting of 8 to 10 tests. I administered these at the completion of every four-week mesocycle. It was too much; there were too many tests. Therefore, instead of good information, I got conflicting results. There was also residual fatigue from the testing, which negatively affected training in the next mesocycle. It was a hard lesson, but one well learned. Two or three progress check tests strategically placed to give accurate feedback are much better than too many tests that give confusing information.

When devising the training plan, carefully place your criteria test and your progress checks in the training year to get the information needed. Testing too frequently does not give reliable information. For example, do not use three tests that test acceleration; pick one. The timing and placement of tests within the training cycle are crucial. Typically testing takes place in the recovery week. Carefully consider the disadvantages of that. The recovery week is just that—recovery. If you put tests in that week and testing is the highest form of stress short of actual competition, is the athlete able to recover? Testing is probably best placed on the first session of the new training cycle when the athlete is fully recovered. This approach provides a more accurate reflection of the training adaptation. It takes advantage of the delayed training effect. Also keep in mind that, depending on when you schedule your test, you will not always see improvement. Explosive tests after a volume loading cycle will often show regression or no improvement. That is acceptable because it is feedback. The testing results reflect the training emphasis.

Certain sports have specific tests that can be used to predict future performance. Obviously no test is completely foolproof in this regard. I have found that predictive tests are only as good as the overall training system. If the training system is thorough and well defined, then the predictive tests are generally very accurate. Swimming typically uses various test sets to predict performance. In middle-distance running, the Kosmin test (devised in the Soviet Union) has been used effectively as a predictor of 800- and 1500-meter performance. I have used a simulation 800-meter test to predict future performance. The characteristic of these tests is that they are part of a bigger picture; they are in the context of the training program. I have found that as my training system became more refined, specific workouts served as good predictors of future performance.

Be sure to include anthropometric tests (the analysis of human body measurements, especially on a comparative basis) as part of the test battery. These tests are useful in determining long-term changes caused by training as well as growth and maturation. For body composition, I have found using six or seven skinfold sites to be most accurate and reliable. It is also useful to take a still picture of the athlete in a front view and a side view to visually track changes in body composition over time. Include length and body dimensions if that is appropriate to the sport. A nutritional assessment in the form of a three-day diet scan can also prove very useful.

EFFECTIVE USE OF NORMATIVE DATA

There seems to be a concern with normative data for comparison purposes. I am not a believer in the value of normative data that attempt to make comparisons outside of the training group I am working with. There are too many variables that cannot be controlled. I encourage each coach to develop normative data for his or her group. When you do that, you are comparing and analyzing your training system, and you control the variables. Over the course of several years, it is possible to gather a large number of test results from your own athletes in order to develop accurate normative data comparing the people within the group. From these results, you can develop a profile of that particular population of athletes. When I was director of conditioning for the Chicago White Sox, the goal of our testing program was to develop a profile of our players in the White Sox system. We tested 150 to 180 players a year with a battery of criteria tests. From those test results I was able to profile the GMQ for each of the positions. I was not interested in how our players compared to other teams; I wanted to test the effect of our training program and track their physical development as baseball players in our system. The tests reflected the control we had over our players. To compare those results to players from other teams who conceivably trained differently would not have been an accurate reflection of our training system. The profile was intended only as an assessment of their athletic qualities, not as a gauge of their ability to play the game.

A key element in testing is to compare intraindividual test results. The most significant insight is to look at an athlete's results from test to test, preferably over the course of a career. The more tests for comparison, the more valid the information. The reason for this is that the only person the athlete can control is the athlete himself. Testing should be a source of information—information about either progress or regression in pursuit of specific training goals. Test to learn the athlete's strengths. Too many times coaches and trainers use testing to identify weaknesses and focus on that. Testing should also be motivational. If the athlete can relate to the tests, then the effort will be adequate to ensure good results. Stress individual improvement and performance relative to previous test results.

PROPER TESTING CONTEXT AND PROCEDURES

For practical reasons, field tests are preferable to lab tests. Field tests, as the name implies, can be done in the field (or court, gym, or pool—whatever setting the athletes practice in). That is where the athlete and the coach are comfortable; it is their environment. My experience has shown that the motivation, effort, and interpretation are much better in this environment. Certainly lab tests ensure a high degree of scientific accuracy, but lab settings must be readily available on a consistent basis to ensure the ability to repeat the tests. Too often lab tests are difficult for the coach and athlete to put into the context of the whole training process. In the same vein, whatever tests that are used should be easy to administer and interpret. If this is the case, it will go a long way toward ensuring the standards of validity and reliability are met. Simply administered tests will help to ensure accuracy. The more complicated the test, the greater the likelihood of error. Ease of interpretation is important so that the test results can be translated quickly into adjustments in training.

Beware of bias in testing. Tests will overlap, assessing multiple physical qualities. This will enable cross-referencing of the various physical qualities. It is virtually impossible to isolate physical qualities since they are so interdependent. The testing should reflect the overall training philosophy. To ensure validity and reliability, you need to standardize everything. A small deviation from protocols can significantly skew test results. Obviously, test protocols should be clearly defined. Be sure that the tester understands the protocol and is consistent in the instructions to the athlete. If possible, test at the same time of the day, on the same surface, and at the same time of the training cycle. If the weather could affect the test, then try to schedule the testing indoors. That is particularly the case with 20- to 60-meter sprint tests, where a headwind or tailwind could significantly alter test results. Standardize the warm-up before testing. Make sure that tests are always administered in the same order.

I have found it particularly useful to videotape field tests. Video will enable you to see how the athlete achieved a particular performance. Archiving this video will serve as a great reference or performance benchmark. Digital video will provide the opportunity for analysis beyond a raw score. For example, in testing a female collegiate soccer player using the Myrland Star Test, I found a .4 second difference between clockwise and counterclockwise movement. In the Myrland Star Test, the athlete starts with her hand on the center cone. She runs out and touches the first cone, returns to the center, then moves clockwise to touch the second cone. The test continues until she touches each cone. After a rest, repeat the test in the opposite direction. Because I had filmed the test, I was able to go back to the video and, using analysis software, overlay the two efforts. This enabled me to see where the breakdown had occurred and work to address the identified deficiency. More important, the athlete could see it and process the information to make the necessary corrections. This is another tool to make feedback of results more meaningful.

The more advanced the athlete, the more meaningful the test results will be. There is a significant difference between testing novice athletes and testing experienced athletes. Testing of younger, developing athletes is definitely a teaching situation. They are learning how to test and how to produce maximum efforts. Therefore, be cautious in overinterpretation of test results in this population until they have had several opportunities to test. With this population I have seen improvement on the second testing date, which I considered an artifact because there was not enough time for training adaptation to occur. The improvements certainly did not reflect training adaptation; they just reflected familiarity with the test. That is fine as long as it is recognized as such. I have learned that single-instance testing does not give the same information on the athlete as when you have at least three tests for comparison. Then you can see trends, and the familiarity with the test and learning are removed as a factor.

There is also a problem in testing an athlete who is not familiar with producing the best effort in a set number of efforts. This is a familiar scenario for the track and field athlete but not for the basketball, football, or baseball player. To ensure accurate test results, I have approached testing protocols differently in terms of number of trials for this type of athlete. Basically the approach is to allow the athlete to test until he or she reaches a performance plateau. Remember that the goal is to get the best effort. Record all the test attempts and note which effort produced the best performance. This will educate the athlete on the type of effort needed and the need for a warm-up. I have found that for jumps, throwing, or short agility tasks, the best result usually occurs between the fifth and seventh effort. I do not use this approach with sprints (anything longer than 20 meters). Obviously this could get out of hand if you are testing large numbers, so it must be controlled. This approach helps athletes learn more about themselves and what they need to do to perform.

THE TESTING PROCESS

Testing is a process, not an isolated event that is an end unto itself. This process must be coach driven, with input from the sport coaches, the conditioning coaches, and, if necessary, the sports medicine staff. I cannot emphasize how important this input is to ensure the relevance and transfer of the testing to actual training and performance. From the strength training coach's perspective the process should include the following steps:

1. With the coaches, determine the need for testing.
2. Select the tests and determine the test protocols.
3. Schedule the tests so that they are logistically arranged in relation to training. This must involve the sport coach.
4. Make sure the athlete is thoroughly oriented to the tests.
5. Conduct the tests.
6. Collect and organize the data.

7. Evaluate the results.

8. Interpret the results for the sport coach and the athletes.

9. Adjust the training program if the test results and consultation with the athlete indicate the need.

10. Determine and schedule the next test date. Repeat the steps in each subsequent testing session.

My testing experience with a professional soccer team in the preseason period highlights some of the essential steps of the testing process. The individual tests were chosen to give an overall picture of each player's athletic qualities relative to the demands of soccer. The tests were intended as a baseline for further evaluation.

- **Testing goals.** The first step of the testing process is to define the goals of testing for the players and coaches. The goal-setting process is done in consultation with the coaches to ascertain what they hope to learn from the testing. I share what I hope to learn; if there are any differences, we reconcile them before beginning the testing. The following are the goals I established for the soccer team:
    - To evaluate the specific fitness requirements of professional soccer
    - To assess agility, body control, coordination, and range of motion specific to the game of soccer
    - To assess strength, power, and endurance specific to the game of soccer
    - To identify movement patterns that could cause injury

- **Test administration.** The testing requires a two-hour time block. This is the maximum time needed. One group starts when the group ahead is halfway through the test battery. Each group will do a standardized warm-up preceding testing. In addition, each player will be allotted sufficient time for his or her own warm-up. All sprint and agility tests are electronically timed to ensure accuracy. Jump tests use the OptoJump optical acquisition system, although many accurate systems are available.

- **Test reports.** A raw test report is made available the evening of the test. This consists of the players' test scores without any interpretation or analysis. A detailed report and analysis will be available within 24 hours of the completion of the test battery. The report is in the following format:
    - The average performance of the group on each test is reported. This enables you to set team goals, such as raising the team average. Tables 4.1 and 4.2 (pages 54-57) provide report samples for general testing and jump testing.

- Each player is evaluated on his or her standard deviation from the mean. A simple way to make these calculations is to enter the test data in a spreadsheet and then use the standard deviation function.
- Video analysis of the tests is available within 24 hours.

Each player's results are printed out on a separate page (see figure 4.2 on page 58). I analyze each player's results and write anecdotal comments. I elaborate on specific training tasks that the player must do to improve the score as well as how and when to do it. I also meet with the coaches to go over the individual results and recommendations. Obviously their input is incorporated and the recommendations are revised if necessary. Then I meet with each player and review the results and recommendations for training. Then we devise a plan to implement the recommendations. I have found it helpful to relate the test results to game situations where appropriate. This helps the athlete to better understand the need for the training recommendations. I prefer not to post individual results for the whole team to see unless the coach wants that. I would rather post the team average to focus on improvement as a team.

TESTS OF GLOBAL MOTOR QUALITIES

The following is a compilation of commonly accepted tests that assess the spectrum of all global motor qualities. Select the appropriate tests based on the demands of the sport you are working with. Be aware that the order of tests is important. You should use speed and power tests early and endurance tests last.

JUMP TEST: *Squat Jump (SJ)*

Measure of contractile strength

This tests the contractile properties of the muscles; it is related to basic strength. This relates to the standing start. Conduct this test with a contact mat and appropriate software.

1 repetition for maximum jump height

3 trials; best score is counted

Assessment is height in centimeters

Protocol

The athlete starts from a squat position with the hands on the hips and executes a vertical jump. Knees must be flexed at 90 degrees at the start of the jump. Landing with bent knees to increase air time is not allowed.

Table 4.1 General Testing Report

Athlete's name	10 m start ave (s)	10 m start best (s)	10 m start ave (s)	10 m start best (s)	20 m fly ave (s)	20 m fly best (s)	
	Right leg		Left leg				
RA	1.84	1.80	1.86	1.83	2.48	2.45	
JC	1.87	1.87	1.86	1.85	2.47	2.47	
TC	1.85	1.84	1.77	1.72	2.36	2.35	
SC	1.72	1.71	1.92	1.85	2.37	2.37	
KC	1.81	1.80	1.92	1.91	2.41	2.40	
RG	1.86	1.85	1.85	1.82	2.30	2.28	
DH	1.88	1.88	1.90	1.90	2.37	2.37	
RJ	1.76	1.74	1.76	1.72	2.20	2.20	
JR	1.77	1.73	1.76	1.74	2.44	2.42	
PK	1.86	1.82	1.81	1.78	2.34	2.32	
JM	1.88	1.87	1.82	1.75	2.38	2.34	
DM	1.77	1.72	1.72	1.70	2.42	2.41	
DN	1.92	1.88	1.89	1.88	2.37	2.34	
CR	1.84	1.82	1.85	1.84	2.32	2.31	
JT	1.84	1.80	1.84	1.82	2.19	2.15	
JV	1.73	1.73	1.85	1.85			
EW	1.78	1.77	1.82	1.79	2.17	2.16	
Best		1.71		1.70		2.15	
Worst		1.88		1.91		2.47	
Average		1.80		1.81		2.33	

Max vel (m/s) for 20 m fly	Illinois agility ave (s)	Illinois agility best (s)	Ajax shuttle ave (s)	Ajax shuttle best (s)	Bangsbo yo-yo speed (m/s) and level	Bangsbo yo-yo distance (m)
8.16	16.05	16.00	10.79	10.73	21/4	920
	15.60	15.30	10.42	10.33	20/6	680
8.51	14.65	14.60	10.05	10.00	21/6	1000
8.44	15.55	15.50	10.24	10.12	20/3	560
8.33	15.20	15.20	10.44	10.44	21/4	920
8.77	15.70	15.60	10.33	10.27	21/1	800
8.44	16.00	15.80	10.71	10.67	19/4	440
9.09	14.45	14.40	9.97	9.93	21/2	840
8.26	15.60	15.60	10.30	10.20	20/5	640
8.62	14.65	14.60	9.88	9.81	22/1	1120
8.55	15.30	15.20	10.29	10.29		
8.30	15.80	15.70	10.39	10.33	21/1	800
8.55	15.30	15.10	10.70	10.67	21/3	880
8.66	15.25	14.90	10.00	9.96	20/8	760
9.30	14.85	14.60	10.11	10.02	21/2	840
	14.80	14.60	10.12	10.02	21/5	960
9.26	14.80	14.70	9.96	9.96	21/2	840
8.16		14.40		9.81		1120.00
9.30		16.00		10.73		440.00
8.65		15.09		10.19		805.33

Table 4.2 Jump Testing Report

Athlete's name	Testing site	Squat jump		Countermovement jump		15-second repetitive jump		
		Flight time (s)	Height (m)	Flight time (s)	Height (m)	Number of jumps	Average height (m)	Power (w)
RA	Pen	0.615	0.46	0.658	0.48	15	0.41	31.16
IB	Orl	0.574	0.40	0.587	0.42	15	0.27	20.2
JC	Orl	0.593	0.43	0.619	0.47			
	Pen	0.546	0.36	0.615	0.46	14	0.37	25.92
SC	Orl	0.59	0.42	0.614	0.46			
	Pen	0.568	0.39	0.591	0.42	14	0.39	29.46
TC	Orl	0.548	0.36	0.556	0.37	15	0.29	22.63
	Pen	0.559	0.38	0.567	0.39	14	0.44	26.73
KC	Pen	0.558	0.42	0.596	0.42	14	0.37	27.13
BD	Orl	0.587	0.42	0.596	0.40	14	0.35	26.63
RG	Pen	0.574	0.40	0.609	0.45	14	0.38	26.82
DH	Pen	0.589	0.42	0.592	0.43	14	0.36	26.22
RJ	Orl	0.593	0.43	0.635	0.49	14	0.44	32
	Pen	0.562	0.38	0.612	0.45	14	0.41	28.81
JK	Orl	0.593	0.38	0.591	0.42	13	0.36	24
	Pen	0.542	0.36	0.557	0.38	13	0.34	22.36
PK	Orl	0.635	0.49	0.613	0.46	15	0.39	31.43
	Pen	0.601	0.44	0.599	0.44	14	0.43	31.52
DM	Orl	0.554	0.37	0.552	0.37	14	0.31	22.29
	Pen	0.546	0.35	0.562	0.38	13	0.31	21.69
DN	Pen	0.561	0.38	0.59	0.41	14	0.35	27.04
CR	Orl	0.258	0.41	0.574	0.40	13	0.32	21
	Pen	0.551	0.37	0.558	0.38	13	0.32	22.13

Athlete's name	Testing site	Squat jump		Countermovement jump		15-second repetitive jump		
		Flight time (s)	Height (m)	Flight time (s)	Height (m)	Number of jumps	Average height (m)	Power (w)
JT	Orl	0.606	0.37	0.558	0.38	13	0.32	22.13
	Pen	0.605	0.44	0.628	0.48	13	0.43	28.69
JV	Orl	0.554	0.37	0.577	0.40	13	0.53	33.33
	Pen	0.554	0.37	0.566	0.39	15	0.31	23.94
EW	Orl	0.562	0.38	0.584	0.41	13	0.37	25.38
	Pen	0.558	0.38	0.595	0.43	12	0.40	29.49

JUMP TEST: *Countermovement Jump (CMJ)*

Measure of elastic strength

This tests the elastic properties of muscle and indicates basic explosive power. Performance on this test relates to 20-meter fly. It would be best to see a significant difference between height on squat jump and height on countermovement jump. Conduct this test with a contact mat and appropriate software.

1 repetition for maximum jump height

3 trials; best score is counted

Assessment is power in watts, watts per kilogram, height in centimeters, reactive index (difference between CMJ and SJ)

Protocol

The athlete starts from an erect position with the hands on the hips and executes a vertical jump after a downward countermovement. Knees must be flexed at 90 degrees at the end of the countermovement. During the jump, the trunk must remain as vertical as possible. The knee angle during the flight phase should be around 180 degrees. Landing with bent knees to increase air time is not allowed.

Figure 4.2
INDIVIDUAL ATHLETE TEST REPORT

Athlete: RA

10-meter left	Best: 1.83 sec	Average: 1.86 sec	
10-meter right	Best: 1.80 sec	Average: 1.84 sec	
20-meter fly	Best: 2.45 sec	Average: 2.48 sec	Maximum velocity m/s: 8.16
Illinois agility	Best: 16.00 sec	Average: 16.05 sec	
Ajax shuttle	Best: 10.73 sec	Average: 10.79 sec	
Beep test	Speed/level: 21/4	Distance: 920 meters	
Squat jump	Height: .464 meter		
Countermovement jump	Height: .484 meter		
Repetitive jump	Number of jumps: 15	Average height: .414 meter	Power: 31.16 watts

Specific training recommendations:

Acceleration work should be practiced two times a week, all with short bursts and an emphasis on good technique. He tends to take too long a first step (see video of 10-meter test). Train maximum speed one session a week if possible. His maximum speed is below average for an athlete in his position. Work agility on the same day as the acceleration work—here the emphasis should be on quick changes of direction and footwork. He should be doing some agility work, specifically footwork ladder drills, each day. His 15-second repetitive jump test indicates good power; in fact, his jump tests indicate good power potential, but the potential does not show up in the speed and agility tests. I also think it is reflected on the field in his inability to gain a step on the opposition. All his work needs intensity. Be as specific as possible and demand intensity. Time the drills where possible.

JUMP TEST: *15-Second Repetitive Jump (RJ)*

Measure of power endurance

Performance on this test also relates to the 20-meter fly. Use a contact mat and appropriate software to conduct this test.

> 15-second effort for maximum height with each consecutive jump
>
> 1 trial
>
> Assessment is mean power in watts, watts per kilogram, mean height in centimeters, capacity
>
> Capacity percentage is the mean height of first 3 jumps divided by mean height of last 3
>
> Capacity: 80 percent = poor, 90 percent = good, 100 percent = excellent

Protocol

The athlete starts from an erect position with the hands on the hips and executes a vertical jump after a downward countermovement. Knees must be flexed to 90 degrees at the end of the countermovement. During the jump, the trunk must remain as vertical as possible. The knee angle during the flight phase should be around 180 degrees. Landing with bent knees to increase air time is not allowed.

The athlete then continues to jump for maximum height for 15 seconds while achieving a knee angle of about 90 degrees for each consecutive jump. The goal is to achieve as many jumps as possible and as high as possible in 15 seconds.

ACCELERATION TEST: *10-Meter Start*

Measure of acceleration

A deficiency here indicates a lack of strength or poor starting technique. It would be best to have as little difference as possible between the two times. That would indicate symmetry starting off both legs, which is desirable in soccer.

> Assessment is time in seconds
>
> 3 trials

Protocol

The athlete starts with either foot 6 inches (15 centimeters) behind start line (which prevents false start with beam). Test begins when the athlete breaks the light beam and starts the clock. Test ends with the athlete stopping the clock by breaking the beam at the 10-meter line. If the test is hand timed (no beam), the athlete starts with the front foot close to start line. Start the watch on the contact of the athlete's first foot across the start line and stop the watch when the athlete's body crosses the 10-meter line. Repeat the test with the opposite foot forward.

MAXIMUM SPEED TEST: *20-Meter Fly*

Measure of maximum speed

This is also used to indicate closing speed expressed in meters per second. This is how much distance an athlete can cover in a particular time. A deficiency here indicates a lack of speed caused by lack of power (indicated on repetitive jump test) or poor acceleration technique.

> Assessment is time in seconds
>
> 3 trials

Protocol

The athlete starts 20 meters behind the start line in order to build up to maximum speed. Testing begins when the athlete breaks the light beam and starts the clock. Testing ends with the athlete stopping the clock by breaking the beam at the 10-meter line. For manual timing, start and stop the watch when the athlete crosses the start and 10-meter line.

AGILITY TEST: *Illinois Agility*

Measure of agility and body control

The Illinois agility is one of the older agility tests currently in use. Its validity and reliability have been proven over decades. This tests the ability to change direction and control the center of gravity. It also indicates body awareness, body control, and footwork. A deficiency here indicates a lack of functional core and leg strength. Any score under 15 seconds is considered good.

> Assessment is time in seconds

Protocol

The standard protocol dictates starting by lying facedown by the first cone. (I prefer to modify the test by using a standing start.) The athlete gets up and sprints to the corner cone, goes around this cone, weaves back around the middle cones, sprints to the corner cone, turns around the corner, and sprints to the finish.

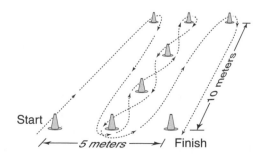

AGILITY TEST: *Ajax Shuttle*

Measure of agility, body control, and ability to change direction

This indicates the ability to start, stop, and restart. A deficiency here indicates a lack of functional leg strength and core strength. A score under 10 seconds is considered very good.

> Assessment is time in seconds
>
> 3 trials

Protocol

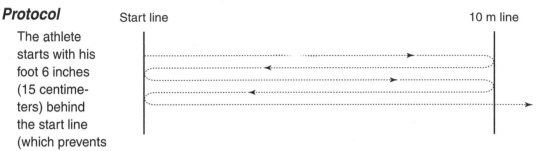

The athlete starts with his foot 6 inches (15 centimeters) behind the start line (which prevents a false start with the beam). The exercise begins when the athlete breaks the light beam and starts the clock. The athlete runs forward and touches the 10-meter line with one foot and then changes direction and touches one foot on the starting line. Once again the athlete runs forward 10 meters and touches the 10-meter line with one foot. The athlete changes direction and touches one foot on the starting line. The athlete changes direction and accelerates forward through the finish line, stopping the clock by breaking the beam. The total distance is 50 meters. For manual timing, start the watch with contact of the first foot across the start line.

ENDURANCE TEST: *Bangsbo Yo-Yo Intermittent Recovery*

Muscular and cardiorespiratory endurance in an environment of agility, balance, and coordination

The test is based on a prerecorded cadence that progressively increases each minute of the test. This indicates specific endurance for soccer in terms of the utilization of oxygen. A deficiency here indicates a lack of overall work capacity. In this test, 1,000 meters is considered the minimum standard for playing 90 minutes at the highest levels.

> 1 trial
>
> Assessment stage is achieved and total meters accumulated

Protocol

The athlete follows a progressively increasing pace over a 20-meter course for as long as possible. At every beep signal, the athlete must have reached one of the 20-meter lines; then, upon hearing the signal, the athlete reverses direction by pivoting on the line and gets to the other line in time for the next signal. If the athlete can't reach the line twice, the test is over.

FLEXIBILITY TESTING

There is a fair bit of disagreement on the testing of flexibility. As Thacker, Gilchrist, Stroup, and Kimsey (2004, p. 372) point out, "Although some persons are described as loose-jointed, a general body measure of flexibility has not been demonstrated, and there is little agreement on the definition and limits of normal flexibility." As a coach I have been forced to use the sit-and-reach test because I was told by medical staff that we needed it to measure flexibility. Once I had the results of more than 400 sit-and-reach tests, I went back and looked at the injuries and performances of those athletes. There was absolutely no relationship between sit-and-reach and any injuries or performance. This underscored that measuring static (motionless) flexibility in positions and postures unrelated to those of the sport the athlete is preparing for is a waste of time.

Carefully observing movement is the best test of functional flexibility that I have found. An excellent daily functional flexibility test is close observation of the movements of the active multistage warm-up. Single-leg squat balance provides much of the information I need to know about any restrictions at the ankle, knee, or hip. The single-leg squat balance is also something that is part of daily warm-up, so it gives me the opportunity to assess an athlete daily. Once you become familiar with the sequence and pattern of the warm-up, it is easy to see deficiencies. The athletes can feel it; you can see it; and it transfers to training and performance. A functional battery of tests that I am now using is the Smart-Test hurdles test devised by Steve Myrland of Beacon Athletics in Middleton, Wisconsin. The hurdle flexibility tests were a collaborative effort between Bill Knowles, Steve Myrland, and me in an attempt to come up with a functional dynamic flexibility test that coaches and athletes could relate to. Most important, we think that these tests can transfer immediately to an effective program to improve an athlete's mobility. This is an easy test battery to administer and interpret. It involves movements that are part of daily training so that the athlete can easily measure progress.

FLEXIBILITY TEST: *Sway-Under*

Measure of dynamic balance, strength, kinesthetic awareness, and range of motion

Body measurements required are overall height and leg length (from iliac crest [hipbone] to floor).

Subject is tested at successively lower hurdle settings until repeated failure. The test result is expressed as the ratio of the subject's height to the height of the hurdle.

Protocol

Align the instep of the inside foot so that it is half the measured leg length from the center of the hurdle. (If, for example, the leg length is 42 inches [106.7 centimeters], place a tape measure on the floor so that the center of the hurdle

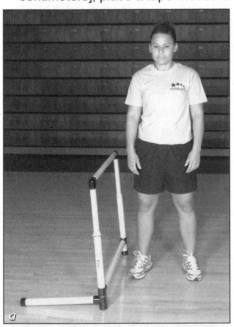

divides 42 inches into halves [21 inches or about 53 centimeters]. The left-to-right sway-under test will begin with the subject's right foot aligned with the number 42 on the tape; the right-to-left test will begin with the subject's left foot aligned with the number 1 on the tape.) The athlete starts from an erect standing position with the shoulders perpendicular to the crossbar of the hurdle *(a)*. The athlete steps through the hurdle opening beneath the crossbar *(b)*, moving from one side of the hurdle to the other *(c)*, elevating to a tall standing position on the other side. The athlete then returns back through to the original side. The athlete must accomplish this task without touching the hurdle.

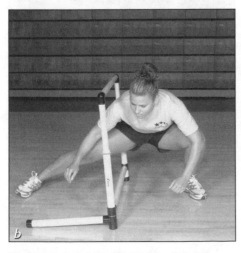

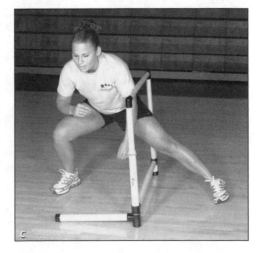

Flexibility test courtesy of Myrland Sports Training.

FLEXIBILITY TEST: *Forward and Backward Walkover*

Measure of dynamic balance, strength, kinesthetic awareness, and range of motion

Body measurement required is leg length (from the iliac crest [hipbone] down to the floor).

Subject is tested at successively higher hurdle settings until repeated failure. The test result is expressed as the ratio of the subject's leg length to the height of the hurdle.

Protocol

This test is done in four parts: forward and backward for the right leg and forward and backward for the left leg. The test requires the athlete to start from

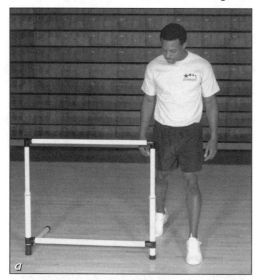

a standing position with shoulders parallel to the hurdle's crossbar (*a*). The upright tube on the free side (the side without the "kickstand" support) should align with the middle of the athlete's body. The test requires the athlete to step forward with the left foot so that it is planted just to the left of the left upright support, and then swing the right leg out, up, over, and back down on the other side of the crossbar (*b* and *c*). The test is then done in reverse. The kickstand support of the hurdle can now be rotated 180 degrees so the same test can be done on the left leg.

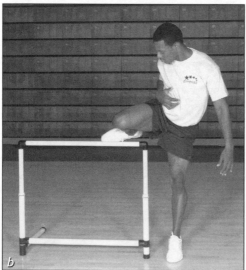

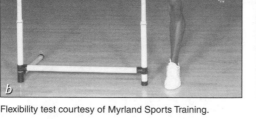

Flexibility test courtesy of Myrland Sports Training.

SUMMARY

A thorough testing program is the beginning of the implementation of a training program. It will provide direction and purpose to the planning and subsequent implementation of training. Testing enables the coach to obtain a good profile of the athlete's physical qualities and compare those qualities against the demands of the sport. Make sure to test all the physical skills; do not take any skills out of context. Based on this comparison, the training is designed to reconcile any differences between the testing results and the demands of the sport. It is a constant system of checks and balances that allows the coach and athlete to gauge progress outside of competition and possibly even predict performance in competition. Remember that this is an information-seeking process. Beware of getting caught up in absolutes. Always factor in the human element: Some athletes test well and compete poorly, and others test poorly and compete well. Keep the big picture in mind when interpreting test results.

Strategies for Performance Training

Effective long- and short-term planning is the cornerstone of the athletic development process. The cliché of failing to plan is planning to fail is absolutely true. To effectively plan to achieve optimal training adaptation, let's revisit the body constant. The body is a finely tuned system of interlocking internal clocks, all of which display predictable rhythms and cycles. All our bodily functions are governed by these internal cycles. The more that you understand and tap into the cyclic nature of the body, the better you will be able to predict and control training adaptation.

The body works on and is influenced by various circadian rhythms. These rhythms control sleep-to-wake cycles, heart rate, blood pressure, neuromuscular coordination, body temperature, pain tolerance, and menstrual cycles. The emerging field of chronobiology can help you guide the training process. Coaches and sport scientists need to do a better job of using chronobiology in planning training.

The most consistently overlooked of the body's cycles is the menstrual cycle in female athletes. This has a profound effect on training and performance, but there is a surprising lack of documented information on this topic.

We have all heard the terms "lark" and "owl" when referring to people who are more effective early in the day or later in the day. This is a biological fact that must be taken into consideration when developing a comprehensive plan. If a person is an owl and has to swim or run heats early in the morning, then workouts must be designed to reset the person's body clock. If the training cycles are in conflict with the body cycles, then the athlete will not get the optimal effects from the training.

CHALLENGES OF TRADITIONAL PERIODIZATION

Periodization is a concept, not a strict model, though it has been portrayed as a strict model. As a concept, periodization is an educated attempt to predict future performance based on evaluation of previous competitions, training results, and scientific facts about the body's adaptive response to stress. It is achieved through planning and organization of training into a cyclic structure to develop all global motor qualities in a systematic and progressive manner for optimal development of the athlete's performance capabilities.

Application of the principles proposed here is more suitable for a sport system that encourages tailoring training regimens to individual needs. Conversely, adherence to a strict periodization model was encouraged, if not required, in the more tightly controlled sport systems in socialist and communist countries, where such training was conceived and implemented along with what many believe was a systematic doping program. To be more effective and applicable, the focus needs to shift to the process of adaptation and the underlying concepts needed for achieving optimal adaptation through the use of a systems approach to planning training. This means that everything must fit into the context of a larger whole. Changing one part of the system changes the whole system. Everything is interconnected. The elements of the system are viable only because of the relationship between the parts.

Planning is essential to sport performance regardless of the level of competition. The traditional focus has been on the long-term plan. It has been my experience that the longer the period for the plan, the less applicable the plan will be. To be more effective, the long-term planning should focus on global themes and training priorities based on competition performance, training, and testing data from previous years. Think of it as the table of contents of a book. It directs the reader to each chapter for more detail. The detailed planning of the microcycle and the individual training sessions is where the focus needs to be in order for planning to be more effective.

We live in an entirely different sociocultural environment than when the concepts of periodization were first articulated and systematized. The following contemporary issues underscore the need to reevaluate the traditional concepts:

- **Decline in physical fitness.** There is a serious decline in basic physical fitness levels and fundamental movement skills at the developmental level. Even elite athletes do not have the broad base of movement skills that the athletes had when I began coaching in the late 1960s. This necessitates a remedial emphasis throughout the athlete's career because it was not incorporated in the foundation. This not only serves to enhance performance but also helps to prevent injury.

- **Extended competitive schedule.** The reality and demands of the extended competitive schedule that exists in many sports today make long-term planning difficult. In classical periodization, the competitive schedule was strictly controlled, and it was possible to plan for peaking for major competitions. Today, because of frequency of competition in most sports, it is much more unpredictable. There was also a defined off-season. That is not a reality today. It is typical for a professional soccer player to play 70 matches in a season. At the youth level it is the norm for a baseball player to play more than 100 games in a year. This reality forces a revision of the classical ideas of periodization. This competitive schedule will not change, so we must adapt the planning to this reality.

- **Doping bias.** Instead of asking if the reported numbers of tons lifted, meters run, and so on were legitimate outcomes of a sound training system, far too many strength and conditioning professionals latched on to the model used in the Eastern bloc countries. The potential to enhance performance by achieving significantly higher workloads in a short period was simply too appealing to resist. But we now know that the remarkable increases in workload tolerance were tied to the systematic doping practices that accompanied the training. And we know that training volume can only be increased gradually for athletes who are not using drugs. Therefore, any legitimate training model should be based on genuine results achieved through natural means.

- **Knowledge of the human adaptive response.** From current research, our knowledge of the adaptive response has increased significantly. We can apply this understanding to various training stimuli, especially in terms of neural and hormonal system response, in order to devise more precise training plans.

To address these challenges, it is necessary to erase the word *periodization* from the training lexicon. I propose that we call it planned performance training (PPT). PPT is the timing, sequence, and interaction of the training stimuli to allow optimal adaptive response in pursuit of specific competitive goals. It is essentially why you do what you do in relation to when you do it. I use the term *planned performance training* instead of *periodization* because it is more descriptive of the process. Calling the process PPT will shift the emphasis away from periodization as a model approach to one based on sound concepts that will work in our culture and society.

SUPERCOMPENSATION

The body is always seeking to maintain a state of homeostasis so it will constantly adapt to the stress from its environment. Training is simply the manipulation of the application of stress and the body's subsequent adaptation to that stress to maintain homeostasis. The adaptation that occurs is fairly predictable. In training the desired adaptive response is called supercompensation.

The supercompensation model is still the most straightforward representation of the training process (see figure 5.1). I use it as a conceptual basis for the construction of my training sessions and microcycles as well as construction of mesocycles. The process is predictable and quantifiable once you have developed your training system.

Supercompensation is a four-step process. The first step is the application of a training or loading stress and the body's subsequent reaction to this training stress, which is fatigue or tiring. There is a predictable drop-off in performance because of that stress. Step 2 is the recovery phase. This can be a lighter training session, a recovery session, or active rest. As a result of the recovery period, the energy stores and performance will return to the

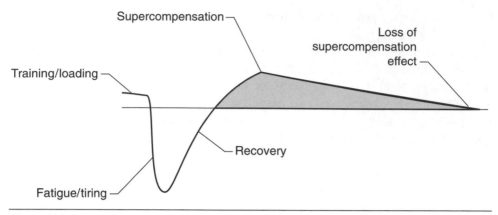

Figure 5.1 Supercompensation model.

baseline (state of homeostasis) represented by the point of the application of the original training stress. Step 3 is the supercompensation phase. This is the adaptive rebound above the baseline; it is described as a rebound response because the body is essentially rebounding from the low point of greatest fatigue. This supercompensation effect is not only a physiological response but also a psychological and technical response. The last step in the process is the loss of the supercompensation effect. This decline is a natural result of the application of a new training stress, which should occur at the peak of supercompensation. If no training stress is applied, there will also be a decline. This is the so-called detraining phenomenon.

Different physical qualities respond at different rates, so it is misleading to think that there's one generalized supercompensation curve. Essentially each physical quality has its own individual supercompensation curve (see figure 5.2). These differences in timing for supercompensation are due to the duration of the various biological regeneration processes that take place during the recovery phase. The replenishment of creatine phosphate will take only a few seconds to a couple of minutes to return to normal levels, but the glycogen-reloading process in the muscle may last 24 hours; in some cases, it may last even longer. The production of new enzymes (proteins) may also take hours, sometimes even days, to complete (Olbrecht 2000). The art is designing these curves of adaptation so that they coincide at the proper time. Working out the timing of the various components is possibly the most difficult aspect of planning. It is as much an art as it is a science. The best way to perfect this is with practice.

In supercompensation the athlete can handle the same training load or a greater load with ease in the subsequent workouts if recovery is adequate and the new stress is timed properly. This adaptive phenomenon is an ongoing wavelike process. If all the variables are manipulated correctly and the proper ratio of work to recovery is achieved, the result is a continually rising sinusoidal curve pointed toward higher-level performance.

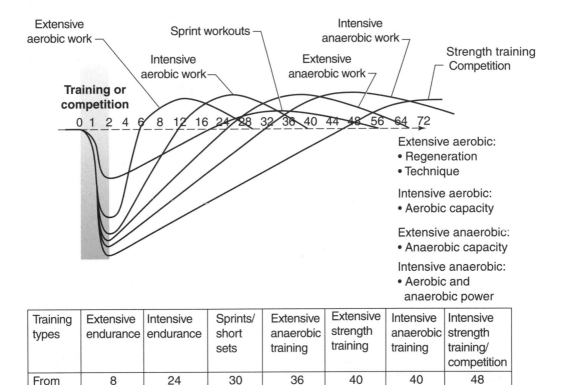

Training types	Extensive endurance	Intensive endurance	Sprints/ short sets	Extensive anaerobic training	Extensive strength training	Intensive anaerobic training	Intensive strength training/ competition
From	8	24	30	36	40	40	48
To	12	30	40	48	60	60	72

Figure 5.2 Time, expressed in hours, to reach the maximal supercompensation for different types of training.

Reprinted, by permission, from J. Olbrecht, 2000, *The science of winning: Planning, periodizing and optimizing swim training* (Luton, England: Swimshop), 5.

To ensure supercompensation, the athlete must be healthy. The training volume, intensity, and frequency must be appropriate for the particular athlete. If training is too intense, the athlete will struggle to get back to baseline, and no supercompensation will occur. If training is too easy, there will be very little adaptive response. If extremely easy training is continued over several training cycles, then the principle of reversibility will take effect. Simply stated, the principle of reversibility is "use it or lose it." If the training load is adequate and the timing of the application of the training stress is correct, then a supercompensation effect will occur.

There is another theory regarding the process of adaptation to the stress of training; it is called the two-factor, or fitness fatigue, theory. "According to the two-factor theory of training, the time intervals between consecutive training sessions should be selected so that all the negative traces of the preceding workout pass out of existence but the positive fitness gain persists" (Zatsiorsky 1995, p. 15). The premise is that the fitness effect of training is slow changing and long lasting while the fatigue effect of training is of shorter duration but of greater magnitude. The two factors, fitness and fatigue, are the immediate training effects of every workout. The most immediate effect of any workout is fatigue, but the long-term effect is the adaptive changes in the targeted motor qualities over time.

The two-factor model has been proposed as a more sophisticated model. I do not think this is the case; rather, it is a logical extension of the supercompensation model. I think that both models are complementary and further explain the process of adaptation to the stress of training. The key to applying the models is understanding that different motor qualities and physical capacities adapt at different rates. In planning training, I use a blend of both models with a slight bias toward supercompensation because that is the model I started with and it has always worked well for me.

PLANNING PRINCIPLES

Training load consists of three interdependent variables: volume, intensity, and frequency (sometimes called density). Volume is the amount of work. Intensity is the quality of work. Frequency is how often the training stress is applied. To ensure adaptation, the body must be stressed to a level beyond which it is accustomed, which is called overload. You can manipulate the overload by changing volume, intensity, or frequency. To ensure a positive adaptive response, you should not overload all the variables at the same time. There is a reciprocal relationship between volume and intensity: If one rises, the other should fall. There are essential principles to ensure that training will be effective based on the variables of loading.

Progression

Progression is the most frequently violated principle of planned performance training. Athletes often try to hurry the process and omit steps along the way or begin at too advanced a level in the training. It is virtually impossible to force adaptation. Progression moves from simple to complex, easy to difficult, and general to specific work. These simple steps in progression give way to complex interactions. All training variables do not progress at the same rate, nor do all people progress at the same rate. Within a career and also within a training year, progression in its broadest sense should occur in the following steps:

1. Basic conditioning addresses the development of the global motor qualities in a systematic manner.

2. The basic technical model involves learning and mastering the basic techniques of the sport.

3. Specific advanced conditioning incorporates more advanced training methods designed to meet the athlete's needs.

4. The advanced technical model refines the basic technical model and builds on it to improve the repertoire of the athlete's technical skills.

Obviously as the athlete progresses through a career, he or she needs to devote less time to basic conditioning and the basic technical model. Once those have been developed, they do not require the same emphasis in each subsequent training year. They should serve as refreshers for higher-level advanced conditioning and technical refinement.

It is important to develop evaluative criteria to assess the achievement of the goals and objectives for each step. I would even say that at certain levels of development it is necessary to show mastery of the current step before moving on to the next step. This is especially true in refinement of technical development. Progression is certainly not linear. Start with a clear picture of what you want the athlete to achieve or look like at the end of a training program, but remember that progression toward that ultimate objective will proceed in a stair step progression. Constant progress should be made toward the goal, but some of the steps along the way will be smaller than others. Factor in the inevitable plateaus and occasional regressions.

Accumulation

Adaptation to the stress of training is a cumulative process, not a one-shot process. A person does not gain an immediate positive training response from one workout unless it is a relatively small technical adjustment. Remember that

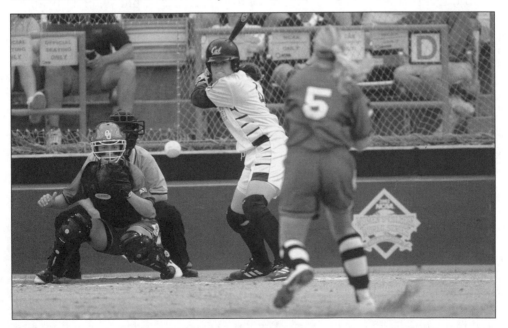

Remember that the effects of training are cumulative; avoid the temptation to overdo the workouts preceding a major competition.

© Rob Tringali/SportsChrome

in terms of adaptation, an athlete is always striving to achieve the supercompensation effect. Often an athlete will not see the true results of a significant investment in training for up to a year after the initial training stimulus.

The effect of training accumulates over time, provided training has been consistent and the athlete has been injury free. Adaptation to different training demands occurs at different rates, and the ultimate training adaptation is the synergistic accumulation of the collective training responses. One workout does not make an athlete, but one workout can break an athlete. As a coach I have made this mistake by putting one last tough workout the Monday of the week of a national championship. The effect was that the athletes left their race in Monday's workout; they were psychologically flat and physically depleted for the championship. Resist this temptation. Be confident in the cumulative effect of the preparation. You cannot make up for something you have not done earlier. Be patient; allow time for training to take effect. Do not get caught up in constant positive reinforcement from workouts; ultimately that will be detrimental.

Variation

The human body's response to training stress is fairly predictable. During the first 7 to 14 days of the application of a new training program, the body adapts quickly. You often see rapid gains in training or technical breakthroughs. After this initial period, an athlete's gains will begin to level off. Olbrecht (2000) terms this the fast adaptation phase. The second phase, usually about three weeks into a training program, is the stabilization phase. At the end of this time the body is much less responsive to the same training stimulus, so the training needs to be modified to ensure continued adaptation. This is the rationale for the lengths of training blocks detailed in chapter 6.

Training volume, intensity, frequency, and sometimes exercise selection must be constantly varied in a systematic manner to ensure continual adaptation because the body adapts to training stress so quickly. This variation should be systematically planned in order to measure the effect of the variation. If no variation is incorporated, there is a significant risk of staleness and eventual overtraining. Variation is mentally refreshing. The following are some of the variables that can be changed or modified to ensure continued adaptive response:

• **Increase volume.** In many ways volume is the easiest variable to manipulate. But I have found that it is not always best to make this the first variable manipulated. Do not get caught in the volume trap because more is not necessarily better.

• **Increase intensity.** Change the quality of work. This alternative is more viable in speed and power sports. For some reason there is a fear of intensity. This variable, although more quality oriented, does seem to put the athlete over the top if it is carefully monitored and controlled.

- **Change frequency.** Add or reduce the number of training sessions. Also consider multiple sessions in a training day to address different components. Sometimes more shorter workouts result in a positive adaptive response.

- **Change workout composition.** Sometimes it can be as simple as a change in rest intervals, or it may involve a change in sequence of exercises. Monotony in workouts can dull the adaptive response. Make sure the variations have a specific purpose and are not just haphazard changes to make things look different.

- **Increase training difficulty.** You can change the environment (such as going from sea level to altitude or moderate to hot climates) or simply structure two hard sessions consecutively.

Any sensible combination of these variables will ensure continued adaptive response. Because there is a reciprocal relationship between volume and intensity, be careful about increasing both at the same time. Avoid falling into the volume trap of adding more runs, more jumps, more throws. You cannot keep adding volume without reaching the point of diminishing returns. The trap also happens because at the start of the athletic development process, volume loading results in rapid and sometimes spectacular gains. In essence, the more you do, the better you get. As training age advances, that paradigm has to shift and the overload has to come from intensity. At more advanced training ages, more volume is not always better.

Context

Context is a key element of a system; it establishes the nature of the relationship of the various components of training within the system. What you do today in training should fit with what you did yesterday and must flow into what you will do tomorrow. The same is true for the components of training. Perhaps the biggest violation of the principle of context is to take one component, such as speed or strength, and train that to the exclusion of all other physical qualities. This is fundamentally unsound. It is possible to design a program in which a component is emphasized for a phase, but it should be kept in proportion to the other components and put into the context of the whole training plan. If the principle of context is not observed, then the components of training will get out of proportion and adaptation will not occur at the predicted level. The best way to keep everything in context is to thoroughly plan.

Context is a principle that I have refined over my years of coaching. Too often a "new" training method or exercise will emerge, and everyone will quickly incorporate the method or exercise into training. The attitude is that if the world-record holder does it, it must be good. The use of chains in weight training and stability balls in core stability are two examples that come to mind. They are viable tools if they fit. Before you incorporate something, you need to see where it fits into what you are doing already, and you need to carefully evaluate the context in which it was successful. Certainly, keep an open mind and incorporate sensible innovations where appropriate.

Overload

The principle of overload is the easiest to apply and observe. It is also the most elementary of all the training principles. In order for an athlete to progress, he or she must be subjected to a load at a level beyond which he or she has adapted. Overload is achieved through manipulation of the training variables of volume (amount of work), intensity (quality of the work), and frequency. Overload is the foundation of the training process.

Recoverability

The principle of recoverability is the ability to recover in both the short and long term from a workload. This is crucial to positive adaptation to the training stimulus. If an athlete is unable to recover from the training stress, then it is not an appropriate load. No two athletes are the same in ability, nor are they the same in the ability to recover. Different athletes have different abilities to recover. To ensure that you apply this principle correctly, give the body the appropriate amount of time to recover from workouts. You may need to vary this time to accommodate individual athletes. Of all the training principles, recoverability is the easiest to overlook because it is easy to get caught up in the work and ignore the ability to recover from the work. This concept is covered more extensively in chapter 14.

Specificity

Specificity involves selecting specific exercises to elicit specific results. An easy way to apply the principle of specificity is to remember the acronym SAID (specific adaptation to imposed demands), which can be summarized as "You are what you train to be." It is more than just doing work. The work must have a specific purpose that relates to the sport. It also must relate to the position or event and be specific to the individual. This principle often causes confusion because it is misinterpreted as training only the actual movements of the sport or the sport itself. This narrow approach will not provide the athlete with the base of preparation and range of movements necessary to overload the system to stimulate continued adaptation. The training adaptation that will take place is dependent on the type of overload that is imposed on the athlete. Specific exercise elicits specific adaptations, which create specific training effects (McArdle, Katch, and Katch 2001).

To effectively apply the SAID principle, you will need to make a clear distinction between similar movements and same movements in the search for the highest degree of mechanical specificity in training. The highest degree of specificity is the actual event or movement in a sport. Unfortunately, this limits the ability to overload in order to improve. You can practice the actual sport only so much; then there are diminishing returns. Therefore, you search for derivatives or parts of the movement or event in order to train the actual movement or event to be better. To make this process more precise, you need to thoroughly understand the biomechanics of the actual movement. For example, it is common to see pitchers and quarterbacks who throw from their knees with the stated goal of improving arm strength. From a biomechanical perspective, this is counterproductive. Throwing involves the whole kinetic chain; therefore, taking large segments, such as the legs, out of the action will interfere with timing and could put more strain on the arm and shoulder than the actual act of throwing would. Another example is alternate leg bounding to improve speed. The goal of this drill is to decrease contact time; but in fact alternate leg bounding results in contact time two times greater than actual sprinting. It looks like sprinting, but it is just similar, not the same. If you understand it is similar, then you will get the desired training response. It will not be the same response as you would get from actual sprinting.

An example of the application of specificity is the use of underweight and overweight balls for the pitcher. Biomechanical analysis has shown that there is very little difference between throwing an underweight ball and

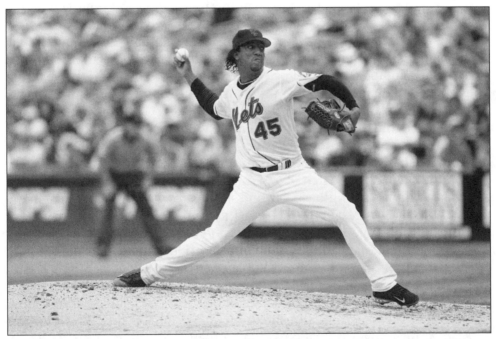

Providing the proper overload for sport skills like pitching in baseball is challenging, but the principle of specificity can help you discover training that transfers to the game.

© Bryan Yablonsky/SportsChrome

throwing an overweight ball as long as they are not *too* heavy or *too* light. Therefore this is a viable training activity that is biomechanically the same for the pitcher. Use knowledge of biomechanics of movement and analysis of the sport to design drills and exercises that will give maximum return for the time invested. The training time will be more effective because it will have more direct transfer to the sport skills.

PLANNING STRATEGIES

In order for planning to be effective, you must implement certain strategies that have proven their worth over time. Clearly define the training goals so they are measurable and observable. Carefully identify key training areas (KTA) relative to the athlete's current competitive status and state of fitness. Prioritize what the athlete needs to work on. It is impossible to do everything. There must be a clear separation between the *need* to do and the *nice* to do. Focus! Do not get caught up in the process and lose sight of the objective, which is preparation for optimal performance improvement with a definite climax to the season or a peak performance when it is needed.

Long-term career preparation must always be stressed so that short-term goals do not compromise long-term development. Training and adaptation are cumulative processes that cannot be forced. Planning will provide constant input on the status of incremental evaluation of progress toward goals. A good plan is like a road map: It enables you to know where you are at all times relative to the final destination. Even though there is a synergistic relationship between all biomotor qualities, they do not all get equal emphasis. The emphasis varies from athlete to athlete and from sport to sport. All components must be trained during all phases of the year, but the proportion changes significantly with training age and the priorities of the particular training period.

Recognize that training adaptation time will change with the particular quality being trained and the system that is being stressed. For optimal adaptive response to occur, some training tasks require complete recovery before they can be repeated. Those are activities of high neural demand such as maximum strength, speed, and speed strength. High neural demand work maximally stresses the nervous system. Exercises of high neural demand are high-speed, high-force movements that are ballistic in nature; they demand maximum effort and concentration. Conversely, some training tasks can be trained with incomplete recovery. Those are activities of high metabolic demand such as basic endurance, speed endurance, and strength endurance. High metabolic activities include lactate tolerance work and work at the anaerobic threshold.

Also in devising a realistic, workable plan, recognize that each training component has its own time for adaptation. Flexibility improves and adapts from day to day. Strength improves and adapts from week to week.

Speed improves and adapts from month to month. Work capacity improves and adapts from year to year. In terms of reversibility, the converse is true. Without emphasis, those qualities decline at essentially the same rate as they increase and adapt.

The physiological, biomechanical, or psychological responses that occur during training are immediate (perspiration, response to training, increase in heart rate, buildup of lactic acid), residual (muscular soreness and fatigue after training), and cumulative (delayed training effect that occurs in the space of a week or longer). If the workout is repeated with adequate recovery, the workout will be less stressful. There is a natural tendency to focus on the immediate training effect almost to the exclusion of the other two factors. No one workout can make an athlete, but one workout can break an athlete. Therefore, the focus should be on the cumulative training effect. Carefully plan the sequence of training sessions from day to day and within the day; also project the potential effect of training on subsequent days. With this in mind, always be aware of the residual and cumulative training effects. The ultimate goal is the cumulative training effect, which is what occurs in the long term. Where does the workout fit in the microcycle? The workout is only one component of the big picture.

When designing training, take into account the concept of stimulus threshold. That is the training load necessary for eliciting an adaptive response. The key word here is *optimal*, not *maximal*. This varies from person to person and with the type of training stress. One of my biggest challenges has been determining each athlete's stimulus threshold. This is especially true in a group-training situation. It is easy to bury some athletes by overloading with a workout or a series of workouts that they survive but do not thrive on. The goal is the cumulative training effect; working at stimulus threshold will ensure a positive cumulative adaptive response.

Consideration of the complementary nature of training units is necessary for achieving positive training adaptations both within workouts (intraworkout) and between workouts (interworkout). Complementary training units are just that: components that work together to enhance each other. The traditional approach has been to consider complementary training units only intraworkout. It is also important to consider the interworkout effect, both between sessions in a day and between days. The following training units are complementary: speed and strength; strength and elastic strength; endurance and strength endurance; skill and speed; and skill, speed, and elastic strength. Ultimately the units have more than a complementary relationship; they should enhance each other and mesh, and the ultimate effect should be synergistic. The simplest means to address the complementary nature of training is to use the modular training approach. Certain units are contradictory. Activities high in neural demand contradict activities high in metabolic demand. In many ways they do more than contradict each other; they offset each other.

SUMMARY

Program design is based on the predictability of the body's adaptive response. Training is stress, and how the athlete responds to that stress is the determining factor in the success of the training program. The planning of the actual training program, regardless of whether it is an individual session or a career plan, must apply the planning principles. It is an ongoing process that will be manifested in the athlete's performance. Chapter 6 covers the actual details of planning and the application of the principles of adaptation.

Program Planning and Fine-Tuning

Planning should be part of an athlete's career from the beginning stages of participation. The plan for a beginner does not have to be as detailed as one for an elite athlete preparing for a world championship. At the beginning level, virtually any work will lead to improvement. Therefore, a beginner does not require an individual plan; a group plan based on biological age can be used. As an athlete progresses, he or she needs plans suited to personal performance goals. At the elite level there is virtually no margin for error; detailed planning is necessary for success.

The key to the long-term plan is to continually assess progress in training and competition so that the plan and the subsequent work are more specific. Olbrecht (2000) makes an interesting distinction in the planning process: The first step in the training process is planning, which involves gathering all the necessary components and data (competitions, evaluations, modes of training, sport and nonsport activities) to improve competitive performance. The second step is training periodization, which involves arranging, scheduling, and adjusting the timing as well as the duration of each type of training and testing for one year according to the fixed objectives.

Sometimes it is easy to get caught up in the process and forget that the purpose of planning is preparation for competition. Everything should be pointed toward the achievement of peak competitive form at the time of the required competition.

LONG-TERM TRAINING

To ensure optimal progress throughout an athlete's career, coaches and trainers need to have command of the long-term buildup of training for the athlete. The long-term plan has four phases: initiation, basic training phase, buildup training phase, and high-performance training phase. Each phase should flow seamlessly into the next. Table 6.1 presents an overview of the training structure for the athletic lifetime. Keep in mind that none of the phases is set in stone. They are very fluid depending on the individual and, to a certain extent, the sport. Sports such as gymnastics and diving are considered early development sports, so the athletes in those sports will begin earlier. Therefore, they demand an earlier specialization and accelerated buildup to high-performance training.

Table 6.1 Training Phases in the Athletic Life Span

Phase	Duration of phase	Stage of development
Initiation	3-4 years	Youth/prepubescent (early school years)
Basic training	5-7 years	Prepubescent and pubescent (middle school and early high school)
Buildup training	3-4 years	Postpubescent (late high school and college)
High-performance training	6-10 years	Adulthood (postcollegiate years)

Adapted, by permission, from L. Sanderson, 1989, "Growth and development considerations for design of training plans for young athletes," *SPORTS* 10(2): 1-8.

- **Initiation phase.** This phase lasts three to four years. This encompasses the early school years. Developmentally, it is usually the period that precedes puberty. This is the time when children are introduced to a variety of sports and activities in a very informal manner. Children benefit most when these activities are playful.

- **Basic training phase.** Typically this phase lasts five years, but in some cases it can extend to seven years. The goals are general physical development, establishing the foundations of sport technique, and establishing training habits and a training routine. The frequency of training during the basic training phase increases from three sessions a week in the first years to up to five sessions a week at the end of the phase. The length of sessions should be limited to one hour.

- **Buildup training phase.** The duration of this phase is usually three years. There is a gradual switch to more specific and higher-intensity concentrated training loads. More emphasis is placed on competition, although the competitions are designed to provide objective feedback on the progress of the training. The number of sessions can be as high as 12 in a seven-day microcycle. The length of each training session is increased. In the later stages multiple daily training sessions may be added.

- **High-performance training phase.** The whole program points toward this phase. In today's high-performance world, with the lucrative economic rewards possible with the extension of competitive careers, we now see athletes competing well beyond what was formerly thought possible. Training is directed by the specific needs of the athlete relative to competition goals. Competition is the focus in this phase of development. The training is of high intensity and much more specific. The number of training sessions is increased by adding multiple training sessions in a training day.

Planning is the preparatory work the coach must do to structure training systematically in alignment with the themes and objectives of training and the athlete's level of conditioning. The process is very dependent on the experience of the coach. In regard to planning, there is not much sport science research to draw on. The training plan should cover all aspects of the athlete's performance. To develop an effective plan, you must consider some basic factors, some quite obvious and others quite abstract:

- The demands of the sport and the position or event dictate all training. Refer to the sport demands analysis (SDA) in chapter 3 for help with this.
- Consider the physical abilities and personality traits of each athlete in order to fit the plan to the individual. Use observation and analysis of test results to determine this.
- Consider the pattern of injuries relative to the event in order to develop a remedial injury-prevention component.
- The "24-hour athlete" concept takes into consideration the demands the athlete faces outside of training. Only a small portion of the day is dedicated to training. What the athlete does outside of training has a profound effect on the training.
- The gender of the athlete is important. Female athletes have different needs than male athletes, which will affect the training plan. Strength training is a more significant part of training for female athletes during all phases of the training year.
- The time frame available to execute the plan is essential. Is it a scholastic situation in which the athlete will be in a program for four years? Is it preparation for just one competition or test? The length of time will dictate the content and complexity of the plan.
- Take into account the specific goals of the plan. The goals should be as detailed, specific, and measurable as possible. Remember that the goals define the target. If the goals are fuzzy, then it will be tough to hit the target.
- Consider the current state of fitness and the current level of technical development of the athlete. The developmental level of the athlete will dictate the direction and content of the plan.
- The competitive schedule drives the plan. Everything is pointed toward improvement in competition. Consider the qualifying format for entry into championships and then consider the championship format.
- A good plan considers more than just work. Athletes need time to recover from the work.

In addition, ask yourself the following questions when developing a plan: What is the performance objective? When is the performance objective to be met? What are the major components the athlete needs in order to fulfill the objective? What means are available to meet the objective? What are possible obstacles—physical, psychological, financial, spiritual, and relationships? Does technique need to be altered? If so, how much time do I need (have) to effect change? What motivational obstacles might occur throughout the year? How many competitions does the athlete need in order to prepare for the championship? Does the work planned suit the athlete in terms of likes, dislikes, and adaptive ability?

TRAINING BLOCK STRUCTURE AND COMPONENTS

The long-term plan is a general guide. It is not detailed because it is meant to be a broad overview of the program. The training is organized into blocks, which are the largest segments of the training plan. It is possible to arrange or rearrange the blocks to meet specific performance objectives. Each block has a general theme and a priority list of major and minor emphases in training. One block must flow into the other without abrupt changes. Think of building a training program as building a structure: The structure is built block by block until the whole is assembled. I prefer the block approach because I can move the blocks around to fit the overall program themes. Once you develop the blocks for a particular sport, then the subsequent programs for that sport are quite easy to develop because it involves simply adjusting and moving the blocks to adapt to the new environment.

The blocks are designated by their specific objectives. The **introductory block** consists of periods for introducing new training methods, skills, or tactics. The goal is teaching, not training! This block usually lasts three weeks depending on the level of development of the athlete. My experience has shown that devoting a discrete period to introducing and teaching new methods or patterns of training will pay rich dividends in the long term. This underscores the importance of getting things done correctly from the start.

The **preparatory block** is as the name states: a time of preparation. There is no competition during this block. The emphasis is on general work to raise work capacity or more specific work to address deficiencies. This block can have a very general emphasis for a developing athlete or a very specific emphasis for an elite athlete. Preparatory blocks are usually six weeks in length.

The **competition blocks** are designed to focus on results in competition. The two types of competition blocks are competition I and competition II. The competition I block is the time for developmental competitions; it is usually six weeks in length. The goal during this block is adaptation work based on what was done in a preceding preparatory block. The competition II block encompasses the important competitions. This is usually three weeks in length and quite focused on preparation for competition. The goal during this block is highly specific application work based on what was done in the competition I block.

The **transition block** is a period to bridge competition and training blocks. This is an active block that allows no detraining. The goals are to regenerate, rehabilitate, and remediate (the remedial work addresses any fundamental deficiencies). During the season this type of block will probably never be more than 14 days in duration. Between competitive seasons it is ideal for this block to be a month in duration. Figure 6.1 provides an example of the block structure for a high-level high school soccer player.

In the training block structure the next step is determining the distribution of work. What follows are the components that are used in creating training blocks. These components include the 21-day cycle, the daily theme, and the individual training session (presented in order from the largest to the smallest component). Each of these components comprises the level following it. The daily theme is composed of individual training sessions (or workouts) and the 21-day cycle is composed of daily training sessions. Thus, if you were to create a preparatory block for your athletes, you could subdivide the block into the appropriate number of 21-day cycles, subdivide those into daily themes, and subdivide those into individual training sessions. This way, as you organize and create the training, you know that every workout is feeding into each of the larger components, which are aimed at whatever goal the athletes need to accomplish for where they are in the season.

21-Day Cycles

A block generally consists of two and occasionally three 21-day cycles. This cyclic structure allows for the distribution of the various components of work that must be incorporated and still allows for recovery. This structure addresses density in a microcycle, the cumulative training effect, the balance of the training components, the balance between skill acquisition and conditioning, and the balance between central nervous system and metabolic training.

Distributing the training over a 21-day period allows a more thorough development of all the qualities and more time to recover from higher-intensity sessions, which has the effect of raising the overall intensity of training. Ultimately intensity is the stimulus that will transfer most directly to performance. The 7-day cycles that are commonly used create a dilemma that results in a tendency to cram too much work into a short period. This can result in a dilution of the training effect.

The six-week block (two 21-day cycles) is not an arbitrary time frame. Olbrecht (2000) has shown this to be the ideal time frame for developing physical qualities to their fullest extent. At the end of six weeks the emphasis must change in order to ensure continued adaptation. The first 21-day cycle is a time of fast adaptation, and the second 21-day cycle is a time of stabilization. Most blocks throughout the year are structured accordingly,

Figure 6.1

BLOCK STRUCTURE FOR A
HIGH-LEVEL HIGH SCHOOL SOCCER PLAYER

BLOCK 1: Preseason

Major emphasis

- Speed and acceleration: short
- MDSA
    - Footwork
    - Change of direction
- Strength
    - Body weight
    - Plyometrics
- Core
- Endurance I
    - Extensive tempo
- Skill

Minor emphasis

- Endurance II
    - Intensive tempo
- Speed endurance
- Testing
- Recovery

BLOCK 2: Fall club season

Major emphasis

- Speed and acceleration: long
- MDSA
    - Footwork
    - Change of direction
    - Obstacle avoidance
- Strength
    - Weight training
- Core
    - Multithrows (medicine ball total body throws)
    - Plyometrics
- Speed endurance
    - ASSE (alactate short speed endurance)
- Endurance II
    - Intensive tempo
- Skill
- Competition
- Recovery

Minor emphasis

- Strength
    - Body weight
- Endurance I
    - Extensive tempo
- Speed
    - Maximum
- Testing

BLOCK 3: High school season

Major emphasis

- Speed and acceleration
- MDSA
  - Footwork
  - Change of direction
- Strength
  - Body weight
- Core
- Speed endurance
- Skill
- Competition
- Recovery

Minor emphasis

- Strength
  - Weight training
- Endurance I
  - Extensive tempo
- Speed
  - Maximum
- Testing

BLOCK 4: Transition to spring club season

Major emphasis

- MDSA
  - Footwork
  - Change of direction
  - Obstacle avoidance
- Strength
  - Weight training
- Core
  - Plyometrics
- Speed endurance
- Endurance II
  - Intensive tempo
- Competition
- Recovery

Minor emphasis

- Strength
  - Body weight
- Speed and acceleration
- Speed
  - Maximum
- Endurance I
  - Extensive tempo
- Testing

(continued)

Figure 6.1 *(continued)*

BLOCK 5: Spring club season

Major emphasis

- Speed and acceleration
- MDSA
    - Footwork
    - Change of direction
    - Obstacle avoidance
- Strength
    - Body weight
- Core
    - Plyometrics
- Speed endurance
    - ASSE
- Skill
- Competition
- Recovery

Minor emphasis

- Strength
    - Weight training
- Endurance I
    - Extensive tempo
- Speed
    - Maximum
- Testing

with the exception of the peak competition block, where the cycles are 7 and 14 days in order to more carefully control loads in pursuit of specific competitive objectives.

This 21-day cycle for a sprinter (table 6.2) is an example of the distribution of work in the block structure. It was developed and refined by Gary Winckler, women's track and field coach at the University of Illinois. The cycle is predicated on training at a higher intensity level and on having a minimum of seven days before repeating the highest-quality efforts.

Daily Training Themes

Daily training is based on a thematic approach. Each day has a specific theme that determines the content and direction of the day's training sessions. The themes ensure that the training and competition targets are met. Essentially these themes do not vary until the athlete enters a competition block; then they are adjusted. The only thing that does vary is the type of training used to develop that particular theme. Table 6.3 on page 90 is an example of a revolving seven-day microcycle for a nationally ranked heptathlete. For example, the theme for day one is neuromuscular accelerative capacity. Knowing this helps me direct the type of training that will fully develop this theme. I know that the work must be higher intensity and

Table 6.2 21-Day Cycle for a Sprinter

Week 1	
Monday	Acceleration development, lactic acid capacity (LAC), mobility
Tuesday	Explosive strength, elastic strength, dynamic lift*
Wednesday	Acceleration development, technical work, mobility**
Thursday	Extensive tempo endurance, general strength
Friday	Active rest
Saturday	Acceleration development (hills, general strength, basic strength)
Sunday	Rest
Week 2	
Monday	Acceleration development, lactic acid capacity (LAC), mobility
Tuesday	Explosive strength, elastic strength, dynamic lift*
Wednesday	Speed development, mobility**
Thursday	Extensive tempo endurance, general strength
Friday	Active rest
Saturday	Acceleration development (hills, general strength, basic strength)
Sunday	Rest
Week 3	
Monday	Lactic acid capacity (LAC), mobility
Tuesday	Acceleration development, general strength, basic strength
Wednesday	Extensive tempo, general strength
Thursday	Explosive strength, elastic strength, dynamic lift*
Friday	Speed development, mobility**
Saturday	Warm-up
Sunday	Rest

*Explosive strength involves jumping with longer ground contact and greater angular displacement at hip, elastic strength emphasizes stiffness, and dynamic lifting is Olympic lifting. The goal of this workout is to open pathways.

**The goal of this workout is to achieve a high-quality day.

higher quality activities that demand more recovery between efforts. If the theme is metabolic, then the work is lower intensity and more general. If the theme incorporates anything regarding competitive demands, then the work is more technical in nature. Always be aware that the themes are general guidelines.

Table 6.3 Daily Themes for a Heptathlete: Preparation Block

	Day 1	Day 2	Day 3	Day 4	Day 5	Day 6	Day 7
Theme	Neuro-muscular accelerative capacity	General and meta-bolic work	Specific competitive neuro-muscular demands	General core stabilization	Neuro-muscular speed develoment	Extensive power output	Rest
Training activities	Speed: acceleration Technical work: throwing Multijumps* Olympic lifts Maximal strength Multithrows*	Technical work: hurdle drill emphasis Technical work: high jump General strength Circuits Upper-body strength	Speed: acceleration (stadium stairs) Technical work: throws Multijumps Olympic lifts Specific maximal strength Multithrows	Technical work: hurdle drill emphasis Technical work: drill emphasis Medicine ball General strength	Speed: accelertion (resistance) Technical work: long jump Multijumps Olympic lifts Multithrows	Intensive tempo endurance Speed endurance Upper-body strength	Rest

*Multithrows are throws with medicine balls, weight plates, or sandbags designed to produce maximum power. Multijumps are large amplitude horizontal and vertical displacement plyometric activities.

Individual Training Sessions

Because it represents the implementation of the long-term plan, the individual training session is the cornerstone of the entire training plan. The individual training session is a collection of training modules. The goal is to facilitate planning and implementation of workouts as well as address the need for complementary training components both intra- and interworkout. The training module consists of specific combinations and sequences of exercises. Each module focuses on one component that should fit with the other modules in that training session. The volume and intensity for the exercises in each module are specifically determined for each session based on analysis of the previous session.

A long-term plan is a succession of individual training sessions done in pursuit of specific objectives. The training session should have the greatest emphasis in planning and execution. Each session must be carefully evaluated and the subsequent sessions adjusted accordingly. Contingency planning is a necessary part of the planning process, especially for individual training sessions.

There is a general theme for each training session. The general theme should be supported by objectives for each component in the training session. The components are very specific and measurable. When planning an individual training session, never lose sight of the most important priority of the session. Make sure the planned session fits with the daily time available for training. Take into consideration the difficulty of the skill being taught if it is a skill session. Make sure the proper equipment is available and that it works. Every component in the workout must be done in pursuit of the specific objectives of the workout and follow the general theme for that particular session. Always keep the training session in the context of the whole plan. A great session out of context can undermine the whole plan. The workout is not an end in itself; it is, however, a means to an end.

In terms of the organization of specific workouts, it's helpful to run through this checklist of questions:

- What should I do?
- What equipment do I need?
- When in the workout do I do the highest intensity neural demand activities?
- What is the time of the training year?
- What is the total volume?
- What is the number of exercises or drills?
- What is the work-to-rest ratio?
- What is the intraexercise and intrasegment recovery time?

Each training session must have a specific emphasis: teaching, training, or stabilizing. In a workout emphasizing teaching of a skill, make sure it is correct the first time. Take time to attend to details and individual needs. Allow more time for individual drills and exercises. The goal of the teaching session is mastery of the skill. A workout emphasizing training is the refining process. This involves more repetition. It may not take more time, but it does demand constant attention to detail. The stabilizing workout is used once the main competitive season begins or emphasis changes in a training cycle. The general theme in stabilizing is to maintain what has been done before. Teaching and training sessions occupy significantly more time than a stabilizing workout.

The key is to design the sessions so that there is a flow from one workout to another. Even though there is a specific focus in each session, the session must be placed in the context of the workout leading into and out of it. Consider the following in the design of each session:

- Sequence of exercises
- Training time available and time allocation for each exercise
- Integration with skill workouts
- Size of the training area relative to the number of athletes training
- Equipment needed and available
- Coaching personnel available
- Number of athletes to participate in the actual training session

Figure 6.2 presents three conditioning workouts for a women's basketball team. This is the last preparation block of training. Not one of these workouts is more than 65 minutes in length. The women are grouped by level of development, which is important in program design for a team. In the overall objectives and theme of the workout, individual strengths and level of ability must be addressed. The best way to do this is to divide the team into groups. For strength training it is beneficial to divide the athletes into groups of three. This allows a good work-to-rest ratio and ensures two spotters if necessary. Look at the overall flow of the three sessions before focusing on the individual components and exercises. The essential training effect is the accumulation of all three sessions.

Figure 6.2
WOMEN'S BASKETBALL PREPARATION WORKOUTS

Monday	
Warm-up	
Speed acceleration	Starts forward, side open, side cross, reverse
Lateral speed and agility	Ladder drills: basic series (with two-foot stop) 　　Forward two-in 　　Forward one-in 　　Lateral two-in shuffle
Plyometrics	Multidirection jump × 4 Medicine-ball wall jump: forward, lateral, and rotational 1 × 5 of each Lateral bound 3 × 10 Hurdle jump 　　Forward 3 × 5 　　Lateral 3 × 5 each side
Strength training	Alternating high pull 4 × 4 Dumbbell snatch 4 × 4 Push jerk (with bar) 4 × 4 Squat (bar) 4 × 6 followed by 10 squat jumps Alternating squat and press 3 × 8

Medicine ball: total-body throws	Over-the-back throw × 6
	Single-leg squat throw × 6
	Forward through the leg × 6
	Single squat scoop throw × 6
	Squat throw × 10

Tuesday	
Warm-up	
Lateral speed and agility	Ladder drills: basic series
	Forward two-in
	Forward one-in
	Lateral two-in shuffle
	Minihurdles
	Forward and lateral, step close
	Reaction coach
	Star drill
	Compass drill
Conditioning	8 × hill (start with shuffle)
	2 × hill backward
Strength training	Incline pull-up 2 × max (feet elevated)
	Incline push-up 2 × max
	Combo I 3 × 6
	Combo II 3 × 6
	Bench press (dumbbell) 4 × 6
	Standing bench press 3 × 20
	Bent row 4 × 6
	Reverse fly 3 × 12 (stretch cord)
	Step-up 3 × 20
Medicine-ball wall throw	Overhead throw × 20
	Chest pass × 20
	Cross in front × 20
	Soccer throw × 20
	Down the side × 20
	Around the back × 20

Thursday	
Warm-up	
Speed acceleration	Starts
	Forward, side open, side cross, reverse
	Then accelerate out and return with plant and around cone

(continued)

Figure 6.2 *(continued)*

Lateral speed and agility	Ladder drills: basic series (with two-foot stop)
	Forward two-in
	Forward one-in
	Lateral two-in shuffle
Plyometrics	Multidirection jump × 4
	Medicine-ball wall jump: forward, lateral, and rotational 1 × 5 of each
	Lateral bound with BOSU 3 × 10
	Hurdle jump
	Forward 3 × 5
	Lateral 3 × 5 each side
Strength training	Alternating high pull 4 × 4
	Dumbbell snatch 4 × 4
	Push jerk (with bar) 4 × 4
	Squat (bar) 4 × 6 followed by 10 squat jumps
	Lunge and press 3 × 3 at each position
Medicine ball: total-body throws	Over-the-back throw × 6
	Single-leg squat throw × 6
	Forward through the leg × 6
	Single squat scoop throw × 6
	Squat throw × 10

Figure 6.3 is an example of an individual session for a developing hurdler or jumper during a competition I block. The theme of the workout is neuromuscular and accelerative capacity. The workout involves seven distinct segments plus a warm-up and cool-down. Two of the segments, the hurdles and the long jump, are technical in nature. Each segment represents a module. The warm-up is longer because this workout follows a day of complete rest. After a complete rest, it is necessary to have a longer warm-up to wake up the system.

An additional block of training for the women's basketball team is presented in figure 6.4 on page 96. This example represents the first week of the competition II block of training. During this block the training will reduce to two days per week. There are also two games per week. No extensive warm-up is necessary because this immediately follows a 90-minute basketball practice. The sessions are both quite short in duration (under 30 minutes). As the workouts progress through this block they will be gradually shortened to 15 minutes in the last two weeks. The faster, more explosive-oriented workout is on Monday following a rest day. The strength endurance-oriented workout is placed on the last training day of the week. This workout is included to help athletes keep an edge of fitness without adding fatigue. The length of this block is six weeks, culminating in the state championship.

Figure 6.3
TRAINING SESSION FOR A HURDLER OR JUMPER

Long warm-up	
Hurdle skill	Walking one step 3 × 5
	Walking three step 3 × 5
	Trail-leg running 3 × 5
Hurdle acceleration	5 × 5 Hurdle from blocks, reduced spacing
Long jump	3 or 4 × full-approach step checks on the track (2 with liftoff)
	Short-approach jump × 6 to 8 (emphasis on setting up the jump)
Plyometrics	Hop 5 × 10 each leg
	Hurdle jump 5 × 5 hurdles (30 inches or 76.2 centimeters)
Speed endurance: hills	6 × hills from third line followed by 3 × downhill
Strength training	High pull 3 × 3
	Snatch 3 × 3
	Squat jump 3 × 10
Cool-down	Extensive static stretching

Figure 6.5 on pages 97 and 98 presents a transition block for a world-class female diver. This block concludes a long competitive season; in the last third of the season she was hindered with a nagging case of patellar tendinitis. Given that one of the main objectives of a transition block of training is to rehabilitate any injuries from the previous season, her main goal was to recover from the patellar tendinitis. The whole focus of this transition block was on rehabilitation so that she would be able to start the preparatory blocks without pain and without any vestiges of the tendinitis to hinder her training.

To further direct the training and stay on task for any sport in any block, designate training sessions as focused sessions or complex training sessions. In the focused session everything is geared to the component that is the focus of the workout; in this example the focus is on speed. Too often, especially in activities of high neural demand, the training effect is diluted by trying to incorporate too many components in a training

Figure 6.4

WOMEN'S BASKETBALL COMPETITION II WORKOUTS

Monday (day before game)	
Warm-up	Medicine-ball rotation Crawl
Strength training	Dumbbell complex × 3 sets Snatch × 3 each arm Jerk × 3 Squat to press × 3
Plyometrics	Alternating rubber band jumps 3 × 12 with box jump-up
Core work	Choose 3 of the following and 3 sets of the exercise you choose: Landmine × 20 BOSU sit-up × 20 Stability-ball kickback × 20 Big circle × 10 each direction Ab roller off BOSU × 10
Cool-down	Partner stretch Hurdle walkover
Friday (day after game)	
Warm-up	Crawls Lunge and reach series
Circuit	(30-second work, 10-second transition, 30-second jump rope, 10-second transition, and repeat) One time through the circuit 1. Push-up, jump rope 2. Squat, jump rope 3. Kettlebell big swing, jump rope 4. Lunge, jump rope 5. Medicine-ball chest pass, jump rope 6. Combo I, jump rope 7. Medicine-ball big circle, jump rope 8. Lateral lunge, jump rope 9. Step-up, jump rope 10. Lateral step-up, jump rope
Cool-down	Partner stretch Hurdle walkover

Figure 6.5

TRANSITION WORKOUTS FOR A FEMALE DIVER

	Daily routine
Warm-up	Miniband routine (band above ankles; keep tension on band at all times) Sidestep × 20 each direction (big step with lead foot, small step with following foot) Walk forward and back × 20 (as big a step as possible) Carioca × 20 cross in front, step apart, cross behind, step apart Monster walk forward and back (wide and low) × 20 (Use early in warm-up and follow it with basic core)
Basic core	(Walking forward and back with 3 kg medicine ball) Walking wide rotation × 20 Walking tight rotation × 20 Walking over the top × 20 Walking figure eight × 20
Hip drop	(Standing on a 6-inch-high box) Front × 10 Side × 10 Back × 10 Cross in front × 10
Spiderman crawl	2 sets of 10 reps
Hurdles	Stepover × 10 each leg
Squat and touch	3 sets of 9 touches
Single-leg squat balance	(Hold 10 seconds in each position; on go to the point of pain)
Hip series	(Alternating days) Series 1: standing Series 2: lying
Lunge	Minilunges progressing to full lunges (add one set a week until you reach four sets) Front up to 20 reps Side up to 20 reps Rotational up to 20 reps
Backward run	6 × 30 meters

(continued)

Figure 6.5　*(continued)*

Additional routine for every second training day	
Trampoline	Balance single-leg squat: Build up to 3 sets of 20 seconds Balance single-leg squat: Have another person run around and jump to create an unstable environment that forces you to react to different movements
Stagger squat	(Every other day) 3 × 20
High step-up	(Every other day) 3 × 20 (10 each leg)
Tubing leg strength	(Attach tubing above ankle) Pawing × 10 (Essentially like a "B" drill: Stand, face the attachment, step over the knee; emphasize out, down, and pawing back) Hip extension × 10 (Stand, face the attachment, extend the leg back while keeping the leg straight) Adduction × 10 (Cross the midline: Stand with side to the attachment, keeping the exercising leg in the air) Abduction × 10 (Stand with side to the attachment, start with legs crossed, and take the leg out—keep the exercising leg in the air)

NOTE: Train three consecutive days and rest on the fourth day. Then, train two consecutive days and rest on the third day. Train one day and rest the next. The rest days consist of manual therapy and massage. Continue this pattern until the next training block begins.

session. Designating a workout as focused or complex allows you to do a better job of achieving the goal of the workout. Focused workouts are usually used in blocks that are high intensity and competition specific (see figure 6.6). Complex sessions are used in times of more volume-oriented general work.

Focused Workout Session

1. Warm-up. This should be very much like a competition warm-up.
2. Power development. This must be low-volume, high-intensity work that will enhance the component of speed development; it will usually consist of multijumps or multithrows to excite the nervous system.
3. Speed development. This is the focus of the workout. This will be high-intensity sprinting emphasizing either acceleration or top-end speed. This places very high demand on the nervous system, so it must be low in volume and high in intensity.
4. Cool-down.

Figure 6.6

FOCUSED WORKOUT FOR A HIGH SCHOOL SPRINTER

Warm-up I	
Strength	Dumbbell snatch throw (12 kg kettlebell) 2 sets of 4 reps each arm Dumbbell push jerk 3 × 3
Plyometrics	Hurdle jumps 3 × 10 at 33 inches (84 cm)

Speed and acceleration	5 × 30-meter block starts (3 to 5 minutes rest between starts)
	   (5 to 8 minutes recovery)
	5 × 30 meters with 30-meter flying start (6 to 8 minutes rest between sprints)
	   (8 to 10 minutes recovery)
	1 × 120 meters with 20-meter flying start

Cool-down	Partner static stretching

NOTE: Speed and acceleration are the absolute focus of this workout. Everything leading up to this segment of the workout was designed to enhance this segment. All the previous work was designed to excite the nervous system.

The complex training session addresses multiple components. This model is typical when using one training session in a day. The daily training sessions in figure 6.7 as well as those in 6.2 are examples of complex training sessions because multiple components are trained. A complex session is effective for developing athletes but not especially effective for elite athletes. Elite athletes have a base of general work accumulated over the years. They will not get as much return from complex work. They need more specific, directed work. The complex session is structured as follows:

Complex Workout Session

1. Warm-up.
2. Technical or tactical work.
3. Conditioning—metabolic emphasis.
4. Strength training.
5. Cool-down.

A proactive approach to injury prevention is to include a remedial component in each workout. The remedial component is based on each athlete's individual needs as well as the typical injuries that occur in the sport. This is most easily addressed in the warm-up. This remedial component

Figure 6.7
COMPLEX WORKOUT FOR A BASEBALL CATCHER

Warm-up	
Throwing	Long toss progression (step 1)
Speed and acceleration	Module I
LSA	Footwork module I
Plyometrics	Multidirectional jump × 3 Restart jump 3 × 5 Restart hop 3 × 5 each leg
Core strength	Medicine-ball power throws (module I)
Strength training	Dumbbell snatch 3 × 6 Dumbbell high pull 2 × 6 Dumbbell push jerk 3 × 6 Dumbbell lunge 5 × 10 each leg (3 sets of forward lunge and 2 sets of side lunge) Overhead step-up (hold medicine ball overhead) 3 × 10 each leg
Cool-down	Partner static stretching

NOTE: Speed and acceleration are the emphasis for this player in this workout. Therefore, it is placed early in the workout so fatigue will not compromise the quality of the acceleration work.

generally takes around 10 minutes. It actually takes on more importance as athletes progress through their careers because they are able to address the small nagging problems that accumulate with advanced age. Make sure that remedial work is done daily, but build in variations because this type of work can become quite tedious.

A well-designed workout includes intraworkout recovery. This can take the form of self-massage, shaking, and stretching. Intraworkout hydration is the most basic and practical form of recovery. Carefully planned intra-workout recovery can greatly enhance the overall quality of the workout and contribute positively to the cumulative training effect. More rest is necessary when the work is high in neural demand. General work does not require as much rest because it is lower in intensity and more metabolic in nature. As a rule, be sure the rest between exercises and drills matches the quality of the outcome desired.

When training a group, carefully plan to meet individual needs. Classic periodization and training theory have not done a good job of addressing this. Everyone will not progress and learn at the same rate. Remember that a team is a collection of individuals, so plan and train accordingly. Carefully group the players in training according to abilities or specific deficiencies that need to be addressed. It is common in team sports to group by position. This is fine for certain workouts but too general for high-quality work; often it does not address individual needs. Not everyone has to do the same thing in training to produce results in the game.

As athletes progress, multiple workouts in a day allow a sharper focus to each workout because the workouts are shorter in duration. Multiple sessions are a necessity for elite athletes; they are not an option. It is preferable to keep the length of the session 60 minutes or less. In structuring a day with multiple workouts, it's helpful to make the first workout very short and remedial, in essence a long warm-up. Make the next session the longest session and then, if it is advisable to do a third session, that also should be short. Think of each session as leading into the next session. Be sure to structure the sessions so that the work is compatible. Carefully consider the ratio of the number of workouts to the number of hours trained. When the hours of training in a week are high, the number of sessions must also be high or there is a significant risk of overtraining.

Constructing a plan for female athletes requires special considerations. Males and females have definite biological differences in terms of strength and body composition. These differences can be minimized with a systematic program. Female athletes, because of lower muscle mass and lower testosterone levels, must have a strength component in all blocks of training, including peak competition. Society still puts limits on female athletes, which can lead to psychological insecurities. At times this conflicts with the competitive attitude necessary for excellence in sport. It can be beneficial for females to train with males. However, in the middle school age range of 11 to 14 years, the biological differences are greatest, so it's not always a good idea for boys and girls to train together. Girls typically mature about two years earlier than boys. During the growth spurt that occurs with puberty, girls should be separated from boys because girls have a physical advantage during puberty. When the boys go through puberty and undergo a growth spurt, then it is again ideal for boys and girls to train together. In fact, I have found it advantageous at the high school level to group training by ability, not by gender.

TAPERING AND PEAKING

The goal of planned performance training is to be at the optimal state of readiness for the most important competitions of the year. This entails understanding the concept of tapering and peaking. Tapering is a progressive, nonlinear reduction of training load during a variable period in an attempt to reduce the physiological and psychological demands of daily training and to optimize sport performance (Mujika and Padilla 2003). Systematic tapering has been shown to lead to an increase in power and neuromuscular function, improvement in various blood measures, and a positive psychological state. All of this leads to improved performance. This process must be systematic and a key part of the overall plan. It is not simply working athletes to the edge of exhaustion and then giving them a rest period in the hopes that they will be ready for competition.

All gains from training should have been achieved by the start of the tapering stage. This is not a time to improve fitness; it is a time to stabilize, sharpen, and fine-tune. The process is both an art and a science, and it is highly individual. There are as many psychological factors as physiological factors in the peaking process. Tapering is about getting an athlete to feel good. This is the culmination of the buildup of training. Throughout the training year you must emphasize that all the training is pointing toward a peak. This reinforces confidence in their preparation. Peak performance is a logical extension of the cumulative effect of the training and competition blocks.

Given the nature of the extended competitive season that exists today, it is much more difficult to achieve a defined peak than when there were fewer competitions and a defined off-season for most sports. It is generally acknowledged by most experts that proper peaking can result in a 2 to 6 percent improvement in performance; of course this is somewhat dependent on the level of development of the athlete. Younger athletes have greater room for improvement, plus they tend to improve more just because they get excited by the novelty of the process.

Some prime considerations are how long athletes can hold peak performance, how many competitions it takes to achieve that, how many times in a training year peak performance can be attained, and whether it is possible to extend a peak. All of these questions must be answered fairly early in an athlete's career. There are no absolutes in regard to any of these. The common pitfalls are peaking too late (usually resulting from a lack of confidence in the preparation) and peaking too early because of an eagerness to get there.

There is a delicate balance between the negative effects of the detraining that occur from the reduction in volume and intensity and the accrued gains in performance from tapering. Training intensity must not be cut in order to maintain the effects of the acquired physiological and performance adaptations. This seems to be true both in developing athletes and high-level athletes. Volume must be significantly reduced. Decreases in volume in the range of 60 to 90 percent can be effective depending on the sport and level of the athlete. The frequency of training must be maintained, especially in technique-oriented sport (Mujika and Padilla 2003).

The time of tapering can be as short as 4 days to as long as 28 days. There are some basic considerations in planning the peaking process. You must have a detailed plan of the unloading (planned reduction in the volume or intensity of the training load) with a daily postworkout assessment. Research has shown that progressive, nonlinear tapering techniques seem to have more distinct positive effects on performance than step-taper strategies (Mujika and Padilla 2003). Step-taper strategies entail planned reductions of training in a step-by-step manner as opposed to a linear reduction. Use only specific recovery techniques that restore and invigorate and do not tear down. Beware of the overuse of massage and vigorous "recovery" methods because they can be very fatiguing.

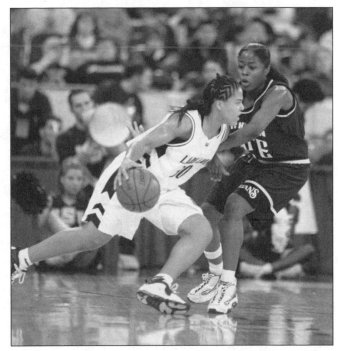

When planning a peak for team sports, monitor the training stress of all the players, not just the stand-outs.

Have a psychological game plan. Increase mental practice during the time of reduced training. Incorporate visualization of peak performance and rehearsal of all aspects of the competitive environment so that when the athletes are in the competition they feel as if they have been there before. This process is highly individual, so be sure to get input from the athletes. Tapering is also the time for their favorite workouts.

For team sports there is very little published information regarding tapering and peaking. Obviously because of the number of individuals, there are many more considerations. The team-sport workload must be monitored very carefully. There is a tendency to evaluate off of the star players, but that can backfire because the role players often determine the success of the team. Therefore you must have a good system of monitoring training stress that accounts for individuals during the tapering process. With team sports, too radical a departure from the players' normal routine tends to have the effect of interrupting the flow. Many coaches think that for team sports it is best to keep the routine as normal as possible.

The qualification procedure and championship format play a huge role in determining the peaking process and the beginning of tapering. Tournament format (whether single elimination or round robin) as well as the team or individual athlete's status coming into the tournament (as an overwhelming favorite or a decided underdog) all have some bearing on the decisions in tapering. With a team or individual who is a strong favorite the first two matches or games can be programmed as intense workouts to ensure a peak for the semifinals and finals. For the underdog, each match, round, or game is the final; therefore they must begin tapering earlier.

It is beneficial to build in a minitapering phase as a simulation to determine how the athlete or team responds to tapering. This should be at least 12 weeks from the planned tapering to ensure adequate buildup again. This is especially beneficial with younger training ages.

The density of the individual's lean muscle mass is a factor to consider in tapering. Very lean athletes will need a bit more time to taper. They also tend to get sorer from the intensity of the work, so increased recovery time must be factored into the taper. Female athletes' tapering must take into consideration the menstrual cycle, because it can have adverse effects on their performance and ability to taper. Some women retain water and feel bloated prior to their period, which can interfere with the feeling of sharpness needed to achieve the taper.

A change in training venue has a positive psychological effect during tapering. With my high school track teams we had a ritual: When we were three weeks away from the state meet, the athletes trained at a better track. It certainly was something they looked forward to. Psychologically it sent the message that the championship meets were different and special. It gave the athletes the feeling of peaking.

Consider the role of competition leading into tapering and peaking. If the competition can serve to sharpen their skills, then it would be beneficial. You should base the decision to add competition on the overall health and fitness of the athletes. Be cautious, though, that any added competition does not distract their focus from the main competition they are working toward. This is dependent on the level of athletes. Athletes must carefully monitor their diets during tapering because a reduction in workload can result in weight gain. Keep neural stimuli up during the tapering weeks—sharpen, do not deaden. Do some workouts to get the athletes tired, but don't program the workouts to have cumulative effects in regard to fatigue. My rule is to get them tired enough so that they sleep well. For many individual-sport athletes the tapering assumes a ritual in which they do nothing outside of their training.

EXTENDED COMPETITIVE-SEASON PLANNING

Team sports with extended seasons are one of the biggest challenges in applying the planned performance training model. Figure 6.8, *a* to *c*, is a model I prepared to address this during the season with professional minor league starting pitchers. This planned performance training model is based on the number of starts in a 140-game season. Most starters get 28 starts in the course of the season. The starting pitchers were on a five-day rotation, which means that they pitched every fifth day. This is the basic cycle of training. The planned performance training model involved setting up a series of revolving five-day cycles. The emphasis in each cycle was determined by the time of the season,

Figure 6.8a

WORKOUTS FOR 5-DAY WORK CAPACITY ROTATION

Day 1: Day after start

Warm-up

Core: Medicine-ball partner rotations × 2 sets

Conditioning: Endurance I

> Start A: 20-minute continuous run at 75% effort

> Start B: Airdyne bike at 65 rpm for 30 minutes

> Start C: Stair climber (level 7 or above) 30 minutes

Strength training: Legs and back (work the legs on day 1 to allow more time for recovery for the next start)

Flexibility: Hurdle walkover and yoga zoo

Day 2: Bullpen day

Warm-up (PNF manual resistance): Horizontal abduction, lat pushdown, biceps, diagonal pattern

Core: Standing core × 2 sets

Balance: Pitcher balance routine

> Pitcher prayer (hold 10 seconds)

> Dip and separate × 10 reps

> Dip and touch × 3 reps at each position: side, front, back

Bullpen: 40 to 60 pitches, working with the pitching coach on perfecting command of a particular pitch or correcting a mechanical flaw

Conditioning: 90 seconds, 75 seconds, 60 seconds, 45 seconds × 3

> Start 1: Run

> Start 2: Bike × 6

> Start 3: Stair climber (level 7 or above)

Strength training: Upper body

Core: Medicine-ball wall series

Flexibility: Partner static stretching

Day 3

Warm-up

Balance: Pitcher balance routine (see Day 2 for exercises)

Core: Medicine-ball total-body throws I (3 kg)

> Stride throw × 6 right and 6 left

> Step and throw × 6 right and 6 left

> Step back and throw × 6 right and 6 left

> Balance step and throw × 6 right and 6 left

Plyometrics: Side to side, ice skater, pitcher squat jump, jump-up

Strength training: Legs and back

Conditioning: Slide board 30/30s × 12

Flexibility: Hurdle walkover and yoga zoo

(continued)

105

Figure 6.8a Work Capacity *(continued)*

Day 4

Warm-up

Core: Wall series × 1

Speed: 6 × 60 yards full recovery

Strength training: Very light upper body

Flexibility: Static stretching

Day 5: Game

Warm-up to pitch: Medicine-ball exercises and tubing exercises

Cool-down: 20-minute Airdyne bike, remedial shoulder exercises (1 set), stretch

Strength Training Components for Work Capacity Workouts

Exercise	Sets	Reps	Comments
DAY 1: Legs and back			
Squat/touch and reach	2	9	
Leg circuit	1		Complete all exercises without stopping
Body-weight squat		20	Fast—1 rep per second
Body-weight lunge		20	10 reps each leg
Body-weight step-up (forward)		20	10 reps each leg
Squat jump		10	
Dumbbell row	4	12	6 reps each arm
Front pulldown	4	6	Close grip
DAY 2: Upper body			
Combo I: curl and press	3	16	8 reps each arm
Combo II: smell the armpit	3	16	8 reps each arm
Dumbbell bench press	3	8	Superset bench press
Rhomboid	3	8	Superset rhomboid
Front cross	2	10	Alternating arms
Swimmer	2	10	Palms out to palms out
Stretch cord routine	3		Do stretch cord routine circuit style
Reverse fly		20	
Nordic row		20	
Pec fly		20	
Punching		20	

Exercise	Sets	Reps	Comments
DAY 2: Upper body *(continued)*			
Remedial shoulder exercises	2		
Prone lateral raise		10	
Posterior raise		10	
Side-lying external rotation		10	
Supraraise		10	
Protraction and retraction		10	
Shrug		10	
Bowling		10	
DAY 3: Legs and back			
Squat/touch and reach	2	9	
Body-weight squat	3	20	Fast—1 rep per second
Body-weight lunge	3	20	10 reps each leg
Body-weight step-up (forward)	2	20	10 reps each leg
Body-weight step-up (lateral)	1	20	10 reps each leg
Squat jump	3	10	
Dumbbell row	3	16	8 reps each arm
Front pulldown	3	16	8 reps each arm
DAY 4: Very light upper body			
Combo I: curl and press	3	16	8 reps each arm
Combo II: smell the armpit	2	16	8 reps each arm
Rhomboid	3	8	
Front cross	2	10	Alternating arms
Swimmer	2	10	Palms out to palms out
Stretch cord routine	1		Do stretch cord routine circuit style
Reverse fly		20	
Nordic row		20	
Pec fly		20	
Punching		20	

Figure 6.8b

WORKOUTS FOR 5-DAY STRENGTH EMPHASIS ROTATION

Day 1: Day after start

Warm-up

Core: Medicine-ball partner rotations × 2 (heavier ball, 4 kg)

Conditioning: Endurance II

    Alternate for each start:

    A: 3 × 5-minute run at 75% effort with 3-minute recovery + 10 minutes continuous stairs

    B: Bike 6 × 5 minutes at 75% effort with 3-minute recovery + 10 minutes continuous stairs

Strength training: Legs and back (work the legs on day 1 to allow more time for recovery for the next start)

Flexibility: Hurdle walkovers and yoga zoo

Day 2: Bullpen day

Warm-up

Core: Standing core × 2

Balance: Pitcher balance routine

Bullpen: 40 to 60 pitches, working with the pitching coach on perfecting command of a particular pitch or correcting a mechanical flaw

Lateral speed and agility:

    Repeat crossover

    Shuttle run (5-10-5)

    Footwork (ladder)

Strength training: Upper body

Core: Wall series (heavier ball, 4 kg) × 1

Flexibility: Partner static stretching

Day 3

Warm-up

Balance: Pitcher balance routine

Core: Total-body throws I (heavier ball, 4 kg)

Plyometrics: Tuck jump, side to side, ice skater, cycle jump, pitcher squat jump, jump-up

Strength training: Legs and back

Conditioning: Slide board 20/15s

Flexibility: Hurdle walkovers and yoga zoo

Day 4

Warm-up

Core: Wall series × 1

Speed: 6 × 60 yards full recovery

Strength training: Very light upper body

Flexibility: Static stretching

Day 5: Game day

Warm-up to pitch: Medicine-ball exercises and tubing exercises

Cool-down: 20 minute Airdyne bike, remedial shoulder exercises (1 set), stretch

Strength Training Components for Strength Emphasis Workouts

Exercise	Sets	Reps	Comments
DAY 1: Legs and back			
Squat/touch and reach	2	9	
Leg circuit	3		Add weight vest or sandbag
Body-weight squat		20	
Body-weight lunge		20	
Body-weight step-up		20	
Squat jump		10	
Dumbbell row	2	12	6 reps each arm
Front pulldown	4	6	Close grip
DAY 2: Upper body			
Combo I: curl and press	4	16	8 reps each arm
Combo II: smell the armpit	2	16	8 reps each arm
Dumbbell bench press	4	6	Superset bench press and rhomboid
Rhomboid	4	8	
Front cross	2	10	Alternating arms
Swimmer	2	10	Palms out to palms out
Stretch cord routine	3		Do stretch cord routine circuit style
Reverse fly		20	
Nordic row		20	
Pec fly		20	
Punching		20	

(continued)

Figure 6.8b Strength   *(continued)*

Exercise	Sets	Reps	Comments
DAY 2: Upper body			
Remedial shoulder exercises	2		
Prone lateral raise		10	
Posterior raise		10	
Side-lying external rotation		10	
Supraraise		10	
Protraction and retraction		10	
Shrug		10	
Bowling		10	
DAY 3: Legs and back			
Squat/touch and reach	2	9	
Body-weight lunge	4	20	10 reps each leg; add sandbag or weight vest
Body-weight step-up (forward)	3	20	10 reps each leg; add sandbag or weight vest
Body-weight step-up (lateral)	1	20	10 reps each leg; no resistance
Ice skater	3	20	Touch the ground on each rep
Dumbbell row	4	8	4 reps each arm
Front pulldown	4	8	4 reps each arm
DAY 4: Upper body			
Combo I: curl and press	3	16	8 reps each arm
Combo II: smell the armpit	2	16	8 reps each arm
Rhomboid	3	8	
Front cross	2	10	Alternating arms
Swimmer	2	10	Palms out to palms out
Stretch cord routine	1		Do stretch cord routine circuit style
Reverse fly		20	
Nordic row		20	
Pec fly		20	
Punching		20	

Figure 6.8c

WORKOUTS FOR 5-DAY SPEED AND POWER EMPHASIS

Day 1: Day after start

Warm-up

Core: Medicine-ball partner rotations (3 kg ball)

Conditioning: 3 × 3-minute run and 75% effort with 3-minute recovery + 10 minutes continuous stairs

Strength training: Legs and back (work the legs on day 1 to allow more time for recovery for the next start)

Flexibility: Hurdle walkovers and yoga zoo

Day 2: Bullpen day

Warm-up

Core: Standing core × 1

Balance: Pitcher balance routine

Bullpen: 40 to 60 pitches, working with the pitching coach on perfecting command of a particular pitch or correcting a mechanical flaw

Lateral speed and agility:

    Shuttle run (5-10-5)

    Footwork (ladder)

Strength training: Upper body

Core: Wall series (lighter ball with one arm, 2 kg)

Flexibility: Partner static stretching

Day 3

Warm-up

Balance: Pitcher balance routine

Core: Pitcher total-body throws I (3 kg ball)

Plyometrics: Tuck jump, side to side, ice skater, cycle jump

Conditioning: Alactate short-speed endurance

3 or 4 sets of 4 × 50 yards at 85 to 90% on 60-second cycle (3 minutes between sets)

Flexibility: Hurdle walkovers and yoga zoo

Day 4

Warm-up

Core: Wall series (light ball)

Speed: 6 × 60 yards full recovery

Strength training: Very light upper body

Flexibility: Static stretching

Day 5: Game day

Warm-up to pitch: Medicine-ball exercises and tubing exercises

Cool-down: 20 minute Airdyne bike, remedial shoulder exercises (1 set), stretch

(continued)

Figure 6.8c Speed and Power *(continued)*

Exercise	Sets	Reps	Comments
DAY 1: Legs and back			
Squat/touch and reach	2	9	
Body-weight squat	3	20	Fast—1 rep per second
Body-weight lunge	3	12	6 reps each leg
High step-up (forward)	2	20	10 reps each leg
Squat jump	3	10	2 sets with weight vest, 1 set unloaded
Dumbbell row	3	8	4 reps each arm
Front pulldown	3	12	6 reps each arm
Day 2: Upper body			
Combo I: curl and press	2	16	8 reps each arm
Combo II: smell the armpit	2	16	8 reps each arm
Dumbbell bench press	2	8	Superset bench press and rhomboid
Rhomboid	2	8	
Front cross	2	10	Alternating arms
Swimmer	2	10	Palms out to palms out
Stretch cord routine	2		Do stretch cord routine circuit style
Reverse fly		20	
Nordic row		20	
Pec fly		20	
Punching		20	
Remedial shoulder exercises	2		
Prone lateral raise		10	
Posterior raise		10	
Side-lying external rotation		10	
Supraraise		10	
Protraction and retraction		10	
Shrug		10	
Bowling		10	

Exercise	Sets	Reps	Comments
Day 4: Upper body			
Combo I: curl and press	1	16	8 reps each arm
Combo II: smell the armpit	1	16	8 reps each arm
Rhomboid	2	8	
Front cross	2	10	Alternating arms
Swimmer	2	10	Palms out to palms out
Stretch cord routine	1		Do stretch cord routine circuit style
Reverse fly		20	
Nordic row		20	
Pec fly		20	
Punching		20	

the league they were pitching in, and individual needs determined by testing and input from the pitching coaches. The motivation behind this approach is the fact that it is a prolonged season. There is virtually no variability in routine aside from home games versus away games. The only place where a variation in routine could be accomplished was in the physical preparation. This worked very well: The pitchers looked forward to the changes in routine, and with the young pitchers we saw good strength and power gains.

The selection and emphasis of work are based on the assumption that pitching is a power and power endurance activity. The effect of training could be easily quantified by radar gun readings and innings pitched. We were able to compare our pitchers to opposing pitchers throughout the progress of the season. The opposing pitchers showed a marked drop-off in velocity as the season progressed. Our pitchers were able to maintain their peak velocity longer, and some of the younger pitchers actually increased velocity. Our pitchers were at or near the top in innings pitched in the minor leagues. Traditional conditioning programs for pitchers emphasize excessive amounts of slow running (slogging), which does not reflect training based on the demands of pitching. The White Sox program emphasized intensity and high-quality work. This program is demanding—it requires intensity, effort, and concentration.

The general pattern of training dictated by the five-day rotation is as follows:

Day 1: Day after start.

Day 2: Bullpen day (approximately 40 pitches).

Day 3

Day 4

Day 5: Game.

There are three distinct cycles, each with a different thematic emphasis:

1. Work capacity cycle has a volume orientation and includes more general work.
2. Strength cycle does just that—it emphasizes strength and strength endurance.
3. Speed and power cycle emphasizes explosive power and also higher-intensity, lower-volume work.

The system was set up so that for each start the pitcher could either repeat the same emphasis or change to another emphasis. The actual season was broken into four phases. The following is the distribution of the emphasis of each phase throughout the season:

- Early season: Three starts work capacity, two starts strength, and one start speed and power
- Midseason: Two starts work capacity, three starts strength, and one start speed and power
- Late season: One start work capacity, two starts strength, and two starts speed and power
- Championship season: Speed and power

This is one example of how to address the demands of the extended competitive season. If a program like this is not used, then there is a severe decline in fitness levels as the season progresses. In essence, the players spend the off-season just working to get back to where they left off. A comprehensive in-season program allows the player to use each off-season to continually build.

ATHLETIC LIFE-SPAN DEVELOPMENT

Long-term athletic development (LTAD) is just that: long term. It is generally acknowledged that it takes at least 10 years or 10,000 hours of training to excel at the international level in virtually any sport. Many people have the mistaken notion that this process can be accelerated, but experience and research are quite clear that it is an extensive process. Key elements must be present in order for the athletic development process to work. First, the approach to development must be athlete centered and coach driven. There is a tendency to adapt adult professional sport models to youth development. This is not appropriate because it is not athlete centered.

Consider that the growth and development process is very predictable, although there are individual differences in the timing of growth phases as well as the magnitude of those phases. Growth happens independent of training, although, given certain windows of opportunity, training can enhance the physiological changes that occur. The most obvious consideration in this regard is biological age. Too often in the United States when training developing athletes, coaches do not consider biological age. Much of the system is based on arbitrary age-group divisions or grades in school. Age-group and grade divisions only serve to accentuate the developmental differences. In a ninth-grade physical education class where all the students are usually 13 to 14 years of age, there is no better illustration of the difference between biological age and chronological age. There will be boys who are over six feet tall (over 183 centimeters) and have been shaving for two years and boys who are five feet tall (152 centimeters) and have not gone through puberty. In this scenario there is a tendency to focus on the more developed athlete to the exclusion of the less developed athlete. It has been my experience that in two to three years when growth and development catch up, the less developed athletes can equal or surpass earlier-developed teammates. If it is a coed class, the differences are even more accentuated because females are significantly more advanced biologically than males in that age range.

Another important factor in the development process is intellectual and emotional maturity. If an athlete is limited in cognitive ability, then you must make adjustments in the structure and complexity of the program. You must discern whether athletes are visual, auditory, or kinesthetic learners. As for emotional development, athletes should be able to handle pressure and take advice and criticism in a constructive manner.

The ratio of training to competition as athletes progress through the developmental process must receive strong consideration. In the United States young athletes tend to overcompete and undertrain; there is a distorted emphasis on competition to the exclusion of training. This just reinforces the Darwinian process that favors the early developing athlete: The strong survive and occasionally thrive. Programs tend to be performance programs, not development programs. Unfortunately, we tend to focus on the few who thrive because they are the stars. The ratio of training to competition must be controlled to allow young athletes to continue to develop through the LTAD process. The youth development teams of the English Premier League in soccer are allowed to play only one game per week. Contrast this to the soccer programs in the United States, where youth soccer teams play in a tournament that involves as many as six matches in a weekend. Which situation is developmental and which is performance oriented? It is no wonder that the dropout rate for kids in youth soccer is quite high.

Dr. Istvan Balyi, a Canadian sport scientist, and his colleagues have developed a multistage long-term athletic development (LTAD) framework that heavily weighs the developmental and biological age in the athletic development process (Robertson and Way 2005). Along with this framework, keep in mind that there are certain sensitive periods in the growth and development process. These sensitive periods are defined as "the periods in human life when the organs and systems that determine a given ability (balance, endurance, speed, or any other ability) are undergoing intensive development" (Drabik 1996, p. 12). During these sensitive periods young athletes are most adaptable to the training stimuli that develop a particular ability. Also note that the sensitive periods are shorter for girls, so there is less margin of error (Drabik 1996). I have modified Dr. Balyi's stages of development based on my experience and input from coaches who work with athletes at these various developmental stages:

Fundamental Stage

Chronological age: Males 6 to 9; females 6 to 8.

Overall goal: Fun, participation, and screening.

Periodization: No periodization, but a structured program with the emphasis on vigorous physical activity five or six times a week.

Competition-to-training ratio: 60:40. (The competition at this level should be informal in the form of play days. Without this reinforcement the youngsters will lose interest.)

Learning to Train

Chronological age: Males 9 to 12; females 8 to 11.

Overall goal: Learning sport skills and identifying talent.

Periodization: Single periodization with sport-specific training three times per week and participation in other sports three times per week. No specialization yet.

Competition-to-training ratio: 40:60. (Competition here can be more formal but must be framed in the context of learning to train.)

Training to Train

Chronological age: Males 12 to 16; females 11 to 15.

Overall goal: Learning sport-specific skills and selection.

Periodization: Single or double periodization with sport-specific training six to nine times per week.

Competition-to-training ratio: 40:60. (Competition should be more formal but must be framed in the context of training to train. Training, not competition results, is the emphasis.)

Training to Compete

Chronological age: Males 16 to 18; females 15 to 17.

Overall goal: Event- and position-specific physical conditioning and specialization.

Periodization: Double or triple periodization with sport-specific technical, tactical, and fitness training 9 to 12 times per week.

Competition-to-training ratio: 60:40. (The role of competition in this phase is learning how to compete.)

Training to Win

Chronological age: Males 18 and older; females 17 and older.

Overall goal: Maintenance or improvement of physical qualities and high performance.

Periodization: Multiple periodization with sport-specific technical, tactical, and fitness training 9 to 12 times per week.

Competition-to-training ratio: 75:25. (This is the culmination of the athletic development process.)

I also like to add to these five phases one last phase of training. This final stage is not as much of a stage as it is a statement of philosophy. It is the stage of retirement. Retention is much more descriptive in what should occur. Athletes, once retired from competition, should stay fit. They should be retained as administrators, coaches, and officials. They have much to offer after they have gone through the LTAD process. The experience they have gained through training and competition can be passed to the younger up-and-coming athletes. They can serve as mentors so that succeeding generations of coaches and athletes can learn from their successes and failures. Unfortunately too often when athletes retire, they disappear from any involvement in the sport, which is a waste of resources.

SUMMARY

The actual process of planning athletes' training is straightforward. Devising the plan is the division of the time available for training into manageable periods. Remember that the divisions of time are not arbitrary; they are based on the type of work that is the focus for that period and the time needed to adapt from that type of work. Also remember to allow for individual variability and take that into account in the plan. Not everyone responds at the same rate. Managing the tapering and peaking processes is a major goal of all training. This is the logical culmination of a good plan. Now that you have learned the foundations of athletic development, you're ready to move on to the actual development of the basic athletic qualities in the following chapters.

Physical Contributors to Performance

 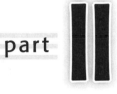

Energy and Work Capacity

Conventional wisdom dictates that, in order to build a sound training program, you must develop a large base of general fitness. There is no question of the validity of this; however, many training experts and coaches confuse building a training base with developing an aerobic base. Certainly an aerobic base is important for endurance athletes, but for nonendurance athletes an aerobic base is only part of the bigger picture. So much depends on the athlete and the sport. Certainly an athlete in a transition-game sport or an intermittent-sprint sport will need more of an aerobic emphasis than a sprint athlete. The real goal is to build a strong foundation of general fitness that has specific transfer to the demands of the sport, position, or event and considers individual needs. I prefer to conceptualize it as building a work capacity base that encompasses all aspects. Work capacity training lays the foundation for more specific and intense work to follow in the later blocks of training. Remember that once a work capacity block of training has ended, work capacity training should not be abandoned. It must be threaded through the other blocks of training in order to stabilize the gains that were made in the work capacity block.

Work capacity is the ability to tolerate a workload and recover from that workload. In order for an athlete to improve, he or she must be able to do a certain threshold amount of work. The athlete must be able to work at a level that is stressful enough to achieve an optimal adaptive response. For example, a sprinter whose general fitness limits her ability to do any significant amount of sprint training would be significantly limited in her ability to improve. Therefore, the goal for this type of athlete would be to build a work capacity base that fits the specific demands of sprinting. This would get the sprinter fit enough to do the amount of sprint work needed to improve her speed.

In the language of training theory, work capacity falls into the category of general physical preparation (GPP). There are three components of work capacity:

1. The ability to tolerate a high workload. The key word here is *tolerate*. Many athletes are capable of doing an occasional high workload but cannot adapt to this workload on a consistent basis.

2. The ability to recover from the workload sufficiently for the next workout or competition. This is closely tied to the first concept. If the

121

athlete cannot recover, then he or she risks overuse injuries or over-training. The athlete will not be able to adapt to the training stress.

3. The capacity to resist fatigue, whatever the source. Fatigue is more than metabolic; it involves the nervous system and mental capacity. Resisting fatigue is the refinement of the efficiency and coordination of the cardiovascular, metabolic, and nervous systems.

In the other blocks, work capacity training can serve as a recovery workout if the intensity is kept low and it is sequenced after a hard training session and before a recovery session. It is usually work involving lower intensity and lower neural demand. It is important to understand the role that work capacity plays in the overall training process. It is more than just work; it is work with a specific objective.

To better understand the concept of work capacity, it is useful to think of it as the components of athletic fitness that, if deficient, would limit the ability to do other training and subsequently limit the ability to perform. Those qualities are body composition, flexibility, aerobic capacity, aerobic power, anaerobic capacity, strength endurance, and anaerobic power. All of these are prerequisites for handling a higher level of work. This chapter addresses the components of work capacity dealing specifically with aerobic and anaerobic work and flexibility. Chapter 10 addresses strength endurance.

Three conceptual terms will help you understand the concept of work capacity. The first is *capacity*, which is the total amount of energy available to perform work. In simple terms it is the size of the tank. In the buildup phase of athletic development, a primary goal is to build a big tank in order to draw on those reserves later. Specific work is directed toward increasing capacity, which is usually volume oriented. The second term is *power*, the amount of energy that can be produced per unit of time. Specific work directed toward increasing power is usually higher-intensity work. The third term is *efficiency*, which is the optimal use of the energy available. In many ways efficiency is the unifying element. Another term for efficiency is *economy*. An efficient athlete has good economy of movement. It goes beyond metabolic efficiency; it also relates to mechanical efficiency. Efficiency allows an athlete to work at a greater percentage of maximum with less energy cost. The result is that the athlete is able to distribute effort over the course of the game or race.

The aerobic base is part of work capacity. However, in sprint sports, intermittent-sprint sports, and transition-game sports, it is not nearly as significant a portion of the work capacity training as conventional wisdom would have us believe. Even in pure endurance sports, I believe that development of an aerobic base needs to be revisited. Keep in mind that training is cumulative. Work capacity will accumulate from week to week, month to month, and year to year. With the aerobic component, once the capacity is increased to a certain level and the aerobic power is elevated, it is not possible to raise those measures significantly. The focus then needs to shift to efficiency, which is how the aerobic component can best contribute to further performance improvement. Ultimately this has profound implications on the selection of the means of training and the actual sequence of workouts.

SPECIFICITY OF THE AEROBIC COMPONENT

It is a given that athletes need to develop the aerobic component. The fundamental dichotomy is how to develop the aerobic power necessary for recovery from the short intense bursts of activity that occur in a game without compromising the explosive power necessary for optimal performance during the bursts. It is during the bursts that actual game performance is measured and decided. This necessitates thinking and acting outside the box. Volumes of research literature and thousands of doctoral dissertations have been written on all the various factors of aerobic exercise. This is because it is a very measurable quality. $\dot{V}O_2max$ is easy to measure; it is still considered the gold standard lab test for measuring aerobic fitness. Remember that what is convenient is not always right. I maintain that, taken out of context, $\dot{V}O_2max$ is an overrated measure, especially for team-sport athletes. I have seen basketball teams put an inordinate emphasis on aerobic fitness tests and be able to run forever, but they don't have the quick bursts necessary for competing in the game. Research has shown that sustained aerobic work will significantly compromise explosive power. For the intermittent-sprint and transition-game athletes whose games demand repetitive sprint ability and quick recovery from bouts of high-intensity work, the effort could be better spent in other areas. Those athletes do not need $\dot{V}O_2max$ tests to measure the aerobic component. Experience and research have shown that $\dot{V}O_2max$ is an unreliable predictor of performance, especially for these athletes.

One of the biggest issues facing coaches who must condition athletes for the demands of intermittent-sprint and transition-game sports is how to train the athlete to recover between bursts of high-intensity efforts. Regardless of whether the recovery is active (as in soccer or basketball) or static (as in hockey), the physiological mechanisms that enhance this recovery depend on aerobic metabolism. That said, the challenge is to train this aerobic component without compromising the explosiveness required during the bursts. There is another vexing problem with this. How do you prescribe the intensity of the aerobic work to elicit a positive training response? The challenge is to find an appropriate instrument to establish baseline measurements to guide the training, and the measurements must be individualized. Traditionally the aerobic component has been addressed by longer continuous runs, which we now know significantly compromise explosive power and do not achieve the desired training effect.

One answer to this training dilemma has been provided by the research of Veronique Billat, a French sport scientist who has shown that in one session an athlete can contribute to the improvement of lactate threshold, $v\dot{V}O_2max$, and running economy. To understand her research, you need to understand two variables of $\dot{V}O_2max$. Those variables are $v\dot{V}O_2max$ and $tlimv\dot{V}O_2max$. The $v\dot{V}O_2max$ measurement is the slowest running velocity that can still elicit $\dot{V}O_2max$. (Remember that $\dot{V}O_2max$ is the ability of the body to consume oxygen at its highest rate.) The time the athlete is able to work at $\dot{V}O_2max$ is known as $tlimv\dot{V}O_2max$. Billat and colleagues' research (2000) has shown that $v\dot{V}O_2max$ and $tlimv\dot{V}O_2max$ are better indicators of performance. Most important, these measures enable you to derive a precise training velocity for the interval work.

To better understand this research and application, you also need to understand lactate threshold and economy. Lactate threshold is the minimum velocity at which lactate begins to accumulate in the blood. It is the point at which lactate removal by the muscles cannot keep up with lactate production, so the lactate levels in the blood rise. The resulting high lactate levels in the blood impede muscle action, so the ability to keep working at a high level drops significantly. This can be seen at the end of a 400-meter race when an athlete ties up. The objective is to raise this threshold to be more efficient in delaying the onset of the rise of lactate in the blood and to be more efficient in using lactate as fuel. The muscles use lactate for fuel. If the lactate shows up in the blood at low velocities, then the efficiency level is low. Economy is indicated by the fact that work can be accomplished at a low energy cost. This is an important measure not just for endurance athletes but for intermittent-sprint and transition-game athletes as well.

The test to measure $v\dot{V}O_2max$ is simple to administer and interpret. On a standard 400-meter track in still wind conditions, an athlete runs as far as possible in six minutes. Record the distance run in meters. To determine $v\dot{V}O_2max$, take the distance run in meters and divide by the time of the run in seconds. The time is always 360 seconds (6 minutes $\times$ 60 seconds = 360). For example, if the athlete is able to cover 1,560 meters, then that would be divided by 360, indicating a $v\dot{V}O_2max$ of 4.3 meters per second. It is imperative to repeat the test every six to eight weeks to determine the new levels. Research and practice have shown that these variables improve quite rapidly. In fact, in Billat's original research using six workouts per week consisting of four easy sessions and one session at $v\dot{V}O_2max$ and one session at lactate threshold for four weeks, she was able to get a 3 percent increase in $v\dot{V}O_2max$ and a 6 percent increase in running economy (Anderson 2000).

As a coach I prefer testing and retesting $v\dot{V}O_2max$ in order to prescribe accurate individual training intensities for workouts designed for developing the aerobic component of performance for athletes in intermittent-sprint and transition-game sports. It is much more practical and efficient. I also think it can be a very valuable measure for young middle-distance and distance runners to be more precise in their training. In addition, I can accurately measure these variables with a practical field test even during the competitive season to assess athletes' aerobic components. The following sections explore the concept further and address the specifics of development of the aerobic component without compromising explosive power. It is certainly a delicate balance that must be carefully planned and implemented.

ENERGY SYSTEMS

When the concept of training the energy systems was first articulated by Fox and Mathews in the book *Interval Training* (1974), it was a major breakthrough. It was presented in such a manner that concepts that had once been the exclusive domain of scientists in labs were articulated in terms that coaches and practitioners could apply. Fox and Mathews identified the energy systems on a continuum of high-energy, short-term ATP (adenosine triphosphate) to longer glycolitic lactate metabolism, culminating in aerobic metabolism (see figure 7.1).

Energy for work can be derived anaerobically or aerobically. The anaerobic system produces energy very rapidly, resulting in large but brief power outputs. But it is limited in the total amount of energy it can produce. The anaerobic system causes a buildup of lactic acid and a rapid depletion of PC (phosphocreatine) stores, which result in a rapid power reduction and a significant drop in speed.

The aerobic system is just the opposite. It can produce large amounts of energy. Unfortunately, this energy cannot be produced rapidly. It is limited by the body's ability to break down carbohydrate and fat with the help of oxygen and, in turn, the body's ability to deliver the required oxygen to the muscles.

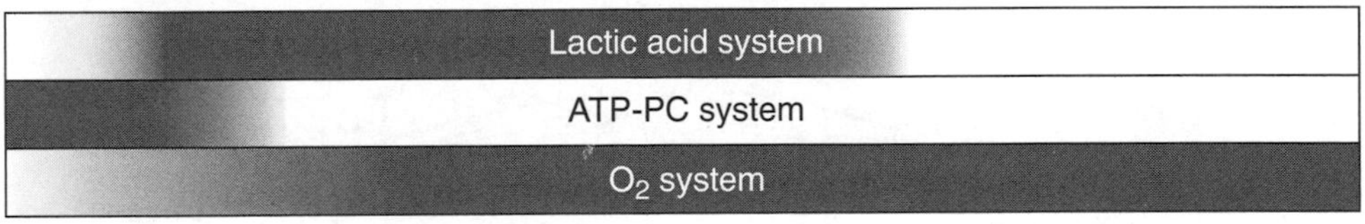

	Lactic acid system		
	ATP-PC system		
	O_2 system		

ATP-PC system	ATP-PC and LA system	LA and O_2 system	O_2 system
Shot put	220–400 yd sprints	880 yd dash	Soccer, lacrosse
100 yd sprint	Halfbacks, fullbacks	Gymnastics events	(except goalies)
Base stealing	Speed skating	Boxing (3 min rounds)	Cross-country skiing
Golf, tennis swings	100 yd swim	Wrestling (2 min periods)	Marathon
			Jogging

Figure 7.1 Energy system continuum.

For the purposes of organizing training and classifying the demands of work, the following breakdown is used: Aerobic capacity is the maximum amount of oxygen that the body can consume in a minute. Aerobic power is expressed as a percentage of the aerobic capacity that can be used; obviously the higher this percentage, the better the aerobic power. Anaerobic capacity is the maximum amount of lactate that a person can produce. Lactate is both a by-product of anaerobic metabolism and a fuel for exercise. Anaerobic power is simply the percentage of the anaerobic capacity that can be used (Maglischo 2003).

Conceptually, the energy systems are intensity dependent, not time dependent. They are presented as a time continuum to facilitate ease of understanding. Somehow the misconception has arisen that the energy systems function as a set of timed switches that sequentially turn on as the duration of exercise increases. But in fact all three energy systems are "turned on" at the beginning of exercise. Essentially the proportionate contribution of each system will vary with the intensity and duration of the effort. All energy systems depend on ATP (see figure 7.2). It is necessary for movement and is manufactured aerobically or anaerobically, depending on the intensity of the exercise. All the systems are trainable to varying degrees. As mentioned earlier, it is most important to focus on the efficiency and interaction of the systems rather than try to target one system for development. You will achieve this by distributing your work in the course of the training plan to match the conditioning demands of the sport with the needs of the individual athlete (Maglischo 2003).

In a similar vein, you will develop the aerobic capacity and power as required within the context of raising overall work capacity. This is all very much in concert with the systems approach to athletic development. No one component is significantly more important than another; what is important is how each component fits into the context of a unified whole for each athlete.

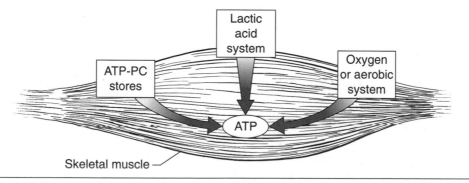

Figure 7.2 ATP is the source of energy for all muscle action and movement. It can be manufactured aerobically and anaerobically with or without lactate, depending on the intensity of the activity.

Reprinted from E.L. Fox and R.W. Bower, *Sports physiology*, 5th ed., Copyright 1979, by permission of The McGraw-Hill Companies.

PRINCIPLES OF WORK CAPACITY

At younger training ages, volume and general work are the primary stimuli for adaptation. With younger athletes, virtually anything you do will make the athletes better. The more you do, the better they get. At advanced training ages, intensity is the stimulus for development. As the athletes progress, it becomes self-defeating to continually try to do more. There needs to be a shift toward more intense work, higher-quality effort, and technical refinement. No component of fitness should be developed in isolation. Perhaps one of the biggest mistakes made in contemporary training is the inordinate emphasis placed on one component of fitness to the detriment of others.

You must work on the careful blend of training components. That is not to say that certain components should not be emphasized at certain phases of the year, but essentially all components of training should be trained during all phases, just in different proportions.

The role of general physical preparation (GPP) changes with increasing training age. With developing athletes, general work makes up the greatest proportion of training. As athletes mature, because training is cumulative, general work assumes less importance. There is less need for GPP and more need for specific work and technical refinement. For athletes at more advanced training ages, general work is used for regeneration and a break from more intense training.

METHODS FOR ENHANCING WORK CAPACITY

To enhance work capacity, choose the appropriate method based on the demands of the sport, the phase of training, the position or event, and the athlete's individual needs. There are various methods of increasing work capacity depending on the sport classification or the specific needs of each athlete. The following methods are the application of the concepts of work capacity. They are the actual application of what must be done to prepare the athlete for the demands of competition.

Continuous Work Method

The most common and preferred method of training to address the aerobic component is continuous work. This work is designed to improve vascularization of the active muscles and enhance the muscles' physical, chemical, and metabolic characteristics. It consists of work in an aerobic zone for a prolonged period. This method is particularly appropriate for endurance-sport athletes (swimmers, middle-distance and distance runners, and cyclists) who are capable of pushing themselves and sustaining a sufficient workout tempo to achieve a training effect. I have found this method to be less effective with sprint, intermittent-sprint, and transition-game athletes who are accustomed to uneven bursts of effort and do not have the ability to push themselves to get a training effect any more than just feeling tired. For example, take a six-foot-eight, 260-pound (203-centimeter, 118-kilogram) basketball forward and ask him to run 30 to 40 minutes continuously at 70 percent of maximum heart rate. It won't happen! Any resemblance to good running mechanics is purely coincidental; mechanics will quickly fall apart and it becomes a plod or a slog (slow jog). The net effect is significantly increased impact forces without stressing the cardiorespiratory system to the degree necessary to elicit the desired training effect. Once again, what is convenient is not right.

The challenge is adapting the continuous method to meet the needs of nonendurance athletes. One solution that I have found particularly effective is what I call the 1/3 workout. It involves picking different modes of aerobic work in order to maintain the intensity of effort. For example, with the basketball player mentioned previously, his primary emphasis is running because it is a primary demand in his sport. Start out by creating a menu of the means of aerobic training available. For the basketball player, you will use the following menu:

- Ground and treadmill running
- Stair stepper
- Elliptical trainer
- Ski machine (such as NordicTrack)
- Stationary bike
- Slide board
- Swimming

From the menu, pick three activities in order of priority. Order of priority means that if the athlete has to run as the primary activity in the sport, then that should be placed first in the work so that quality is ensured in the primary activity. After that, the criterion for choosing the activities is to go from highest impact to lowest impact. Determine a target for total training time, such as 30 minutes. Then divide that time period into thirds. The first 10 minutes is a run. Then immediately switch to the next preferable mode, such as stair stepper, for 10 minutes. At the completion of that, go to the third, the lowest-impact method, such as the slide board, for 10 minutes. This enables the athlete to complete 30 minutes of continuous work at a higher-intensity effort than if he would have run for 30 minutes. It is not perfect, but it works. Keep in mind that this will not produce a high-level 10K runner, but it will enable athletes not accustomed to prolonged running or those who are unable to push themselves to get a very beneficial aerobic training effect. It is a means to an end.

Variation Method

The second method of work capacity development is the variation method. This is also called *fartlek*, which is the Swedish word for *speed play*. I like to think of this method as high-level game or race simulation. It is essentially a continuous workout in which intensity is varied throughout until the target time of the workout is reached. Various activities occur in different combinations and at varied intensities to make up all the movements of the game. The variation method affords the opportunity to incorporate all those varied movements and intensities into a workout that will simulate the demands of the game. The workout can be designed to be more specific to positions or to how an athlete plays the game. The variation method can be very structured or loosely structured depending on the objective. It can be inner directed (driven by the athlete) or structured to respond to demands from the coach to perform various activities throughout the workout. For nonendurance athletes, one fartlek workout in a seven-day microcycle for a maximum of six workouts is sufficient for achieving the desired training response. For endurance athletes, this is a great workout to simulate the various changes of pace that occur throughout the race. It is a race-hardening workout.

The following is an example of a variation workout for soccer. I call it the *smorgy* to describe the variety of activities that are incorporated. This particular workout was a game-hardening workout done late in the preparation phase for a professional soccer player. It was placed on Saturday, the sixth day of a training week, when cumulative fatigue was highest to achieve a game-simulation effect. It consists of six segments done continuously. The runs should involve curves, angles, and cuts. The goal is to simulate the demands of the game, and in the game very little running is straight ahead.

1. 15/15/15 runs. 15-second walk, 15-second run, 15-second sprint × 6 sets.
2. 10-second bursts (30 seconds easy jog recovery) × 10.
3. Short/short/long × 10 reps. Two short touches with the ball followed by a longer touch; sprint after the ball. Easy dribbles for 30 seconds of recovery and repeat.
4. 1-minute shuttle (20 meters—as many reps as possible in the minute).
5. 30 seconds of juggling, then sprint 10 yards; repeat five times.
6. One versus one with passive defense (in penalty area); three touches and a shot, then sprint to midfield. Jog back for recovery. Repeat five times.

Another way to structure fartlek workouts that is less movement specific but still very demanding metabolically is to pick a target time that you would like your athletes to achieve in the fartlek workout (for example,

20 minutes). Then devise a logical progression to get the athletes to that time goal. Assign a specific number of hard efforts for each time period. For example, use 10 efforts between 30 and 90 seconds in 20 minutes, then let each athlete determine the actual distribution. This allows you to control the density of the workout but the athletes can control the intensity. I have found that it takes a more mature athlete with a good work capacity to get a good training effect from this method. For less mature athletes or team-sport athletes, "whistle fartlek" is especially effective. The procedure is the same, but the coach blows a whistle to begin the hard effort and then blows the whistle again to signal the end of a hard effort until the number of hard efforts in the target time is reached.

Interval Method

The third method of work capacity development is the interval method. In many ways this is the most effective and applicable method for the non-endurance athlete. It is very quantifiable and can be made very specific. It is the best method for developing an aerobic component with a minimal sacrifice of explosiveness. As the name implies, in this method of training the focus is on the interval of work and rest. By manipulating the length, duration, or intensity of the interval relative to the length of the rest interval, the training effect can be significantly altered. I break interval training into two classifications adapted from the work of Gerard Mach, former national track and field coach of Canada. Rather than base the intervals on heart rate, I choose to use perceived exertion. I have found that teaching the athletes to tune in to their bodies by learning a percentage of maximum effort has a very good carryover to their sports.

When I began coaching I was exposed to what later became known as a rating of perceived exertion scale. Mihaly Igloi, the Hungarian middle-distance and long-distance coach whose training system was based on interval training, based the intensity of interval work on descriptors of effort (Mulak 1964). I find this approach easy to use with the athletes and very effective at getting them to tune in to their bodies and feel the effort required to run workouts of varied effort. These descriptors are basically a scale of perceived exertion. The gradations are progressive, leading up to all-out race effort.

Easy: Used for recovery.

Medium easy: Moderate effort.

Medium: A little harder, but still conversational.

Swing: Fast but still controlled; you should still feel as if you have another gear.

Fast: Just as the name implies.

Race: Highest effort.

This is a method of getting runners to tune in to their bodies and feel the effort required by the particular interval. I find this to be an especially effective system in helping athletes to learn the feel and the rhythm of the required effort.

Extensive Tempo Intervals

The first classification of interval training is extensive tempo intervals (ETE). This consists of work at 80 percent or less of maximum effort. This is essentially aerobic interval work. This is the type of work that should be the focus for soccer, basketball, lacrosse, or field hockey players who want to improve aerobic capacity and power. The simplest extensive interval workout is repeated 100-meter runs with 30 seconds of rest. Over the years this has proven to be an effective way to reinforce correct running mechanics and still get a good aerobic training effect. A relatively unfit athlete can manage 100 meters (110 yards) with good rhythm and running mechanics. The distance–time relationship allows athletes to maintain a solid effort even when they are starting a program at a low level of work capacity. The key to this workout is an athlete's ability to hold the rest interval while maintaining the pace of the runs.

Extensive Interval Workout: 100-Meter Runs

Week 1: 16 × 100 meters in 22 seconds; 30 seconds of rest between runs.

Week 2: 18 × 100 meters in 22 seconds; 30 seconds of rest between runs.

Week 3: 16 × 100 meters in 21 seconds; 30 seconds of rest between runs.

Week 4: 18 × 100 meters in 21 seconds; 45 seconds of rest between runs.

Week 5: 16 × 100 meters in 20 seconds; 45 seconds of rest between runs.

Week 6: 18 × 100 meters in 20 seconds; 45 seconds of rest between runs.

The workout is performed once every seven days until the progression is accomplished.

Another effective extensive interval workout for improving $\dot{V}O_2$max is the 30/30 workout. This workout can significantly raise $\dot{V}O_2$max. As Veronique Billat has shown, this particular work-to-rest interval done at $v\dot{V}O_2$ will raise $\dot{V}O_2$max, raise the lactate threshold, and improve running economy. I have found this workout to be quite effective in raising fitness levels if used once a week for six weeks. This simply consists of a 30-second run at 70 percent effort followed by 30 seconds of recovery. The recovery can be a walk or a jog. This workout can be easily adapted to modes other than running, such as slide board or bike. If you use a bike, add about 25 percent more repetitions.

If you so desire, you can use Billat's $v\dot{V}O_2max$ six-minute run test to determine a specific distance to run for the 30 seconds and then you can run the recovery 30 seconds at 50 percent $v\dot{V}O_2max$. From the previous example, the athlete who covered 1,560 meters in the six-minute test had a $v\dot{V}O_2max$ of 4.3 meters per second; then the athlete would run 130 meters in 30 seconds and 65 meters during the recovery 30 seconds. This figure is derived by multiplying the $v\dot{V}O_2max$ by 30 seconds. I have not used this approach on the 30/30 workout because it does not lend itself well to a group setting, so it is not very practical to use with a team. I prefer to teach athletes the feel of effort by using Igloi's terms because it has better carryover to the game or race.

Extensive Interval Workout: 30/30 Workout

Week 1: 12 × 30-second run/30-second walk.

Week 2: 15 × 30-second run/30-second jog.

Week 3: 18 × 30-second run/30-second jog.

Week 4: 21 × 30-second run/30-second jog.

Week 5: 24 × 30-second run/30-second jog.

Week 6: 27 × 30-second run/30-second jog.

The time of 30 seconds is one in which a nonendurance athlete can cover a decent distance and be able to recover in the subsequent 30 seconds to keep reproducing the required effort. A good perimeter player in high school basketball should be able to do 21 to 24 reps of this to be considered fit to play. A post player at the same level should be able to do 18 to 21 repetitions. A professional soccer midfield player should be able to do 30 repetitions at 75 percent. This is a workout I have used for years. It is best placed in the general preparation foundation block of training, although it can be effective to bring it back occasionally in the early competition block.

Intensive Tempo Endurance

The second classification of interval training is intensive tempo endurance (ITE). This consists of work between 80 and 90 percent of maximum effort. It is a mix of aerobic and anaerobic work. The work is very taxing and results in significant residual fatigue if overused. It is usually used in a ratio of approximately one intensive interval session to every three or four extensive interval sessions.

One intensive tempo endurance workout is the staircase 30s plus max run. This workout addresses the spectrum from sustained aerobic to anaerobic lactate production work. It is a very good workout for the intermittent- and transition-game athlete during a special preparation block of training. This requires a buildup of effort as the workout proceeds. The objective is to teach athletes to manage the fatigue, not let it manage them. Accomplishing this requires increasing effort in order to maintain pace. You learn to go faster when you are tired!

Intensive Tempo Endurance Workout: Staircase 30s Plus Max Run

45 seconds recovery after 30-second runs, 30-second runs at increasing effort:

1 × 70 percent, 1 × 75 percent, 1 × 80 percent, plus 3-minute run at maximum effort; 3-minute jog recovery.

1 × 75 percent, 1 × 80 percent, 1 × 85 percent, plus 2-minute run at maximum effort; 3-minute jog recovery.

1 × 80 percent, 1 × 85 percent, 1 × 90 percent, plus 1-minute run at maximum effort.

Another intensive tempo endurance workout is the 15/15/15 workout. This workout is appropriate in an early competition block. The workout was inspired by the research of Billat and colleagues (2001).

Intensive Tempo Endurance Workout: 15/15/15 Workout

15-second walk, 15-second run at 80 percent, 15-second sprint at 90 percent; 9 reps in week 1; 12 reps in week 2; 15 reps in week 3.

Repetition Method

The most demanding and intense work capacity method is the repetition method, which is used for improving economy of effort. It is characterized by a high-intensity workload alternated with complete rest to allow for full recovery between repetitions. It is also called special endurance. The work is in a range of 90 to 100 percent effort. An example is a 45-second all-out run for distance with 15 to 20 minutes of recovery, followed by another 45-second run all out for distance. Compare the distance of the two runs to evaluate the workout. From track and field, 3 × 200 meters at 95 percent intensity with 15 minutes of recovery is another example of the repetition method. The repetition method sharpens and prepares athletes for specific competitive efforts. The volume is very low and the intensity is very high. Repetition work is done at race effort.

Cross-Training Method

Cross-training is a term that has gained fairly wide acceptance in training in the last 15 years. Cross-training involves training in a discipline other than the main sport for the sole purpose of enhancing performance in the primary event (Hawley and Burke 1998). The origin of the term probably lies with the first triathletes. It has been used as a method for retaining training adaptations during times of injury, but it has also been used as a supplementary training method for raising work capacity. What you must be aware of is transfer of training effect. My experience has shown that those who use cross-training already have a tendency to chronically overwork and are looking for another way to add more work. The concept of cross-training is another training myth that has actually detracted from sound training. It certainly has very little foundation in sport science research. For a runner to get in the pool for anything more than a recovery session is time ill spent. The same is true of biking for a runner: That time would be better spent strength training or working on flexibility, areas that tend to be ignored because runners often think they do not have enough time to fit these modes into their overall training. Yet those same runners can find the time to swim for 30 minutes or bike for 60 minutes. It is all a matter of priorities.

Research does seem to indicate that there is more transfer of training effect from cycling to running than from running to cycling. In other words, cycling will help runners more than running will help cyclists. My experience as a coach certainly has borne this out. Cross-training can be beneficial for recreational athletes seeking to raise general fitness or relieve the boredom of training, but for high-level athletes the returns are not commensurate with the time invested. Specific exercise elicits specific adaptations, creating specific training effects (McArdle, Katch, and Katch 2001). For performance and aerobic benefit, cross-training using disparate methods would be effective only for participants of lower aerobic capacity. Well-trained people derive more benefit from cross-training with the use of similar modes (Loy, Hoffmann, and Holland 1995). Keep in mind that a comprehensive training program incorporates a variety of means for achieving various training goals. So it is imperative to have a specific purpose for choosing different modes of training.

SAMPLE WORK CAPACITY BLOCK

Figure 7.3 is an example of a six-week foundation block of training for a men's collegiate soccer team. The emphasis here is on raising work capacity, especially aerobic power.

This is the first block of the summer training. Because the players are not in school, the work is unsupervised. The players receive the program and are expected to do it on their own. The assumption is that they will all be playing on teams during the summer or will be doing something soccer specific at least five days per week in addition to the conditioning program. In the structure of the collegiate system, this block has the biggest emphasis on endurance and work capacity. This realistically is the only block during the year when that could be emphasized without compromising the development of other qualities. The previous block emphasized speed and explosive power. That was done so that work that had a higher technical demand could be supervised. This also reflects the principle of speed before speed endurance and strength before strength endurance.

Figure 7.3

SAMPLE WORK CAPACITY BLOCK

WEEK 1	Theme: Reestablish routine
Monday	1 × 10-minute run at 70 percent; 5-minute recovery; 3 × 5-minute runs at 75 percent; 3-minute recovery between runs
Tuesday	20 × 30/30 at 75 percent Strength training: total body
Wednesday	Active rest
Thursday	8 minutes of continuous hills + 5 minutes of hard run Strength training: total body
Friday	6 × 2-minute runs at 85 percent with 3-minute walking recovery
Saturday	30-minute steady run at 70 percent effort of game
Sunday	Rest

NOTE: Thursday's workout is designed to develop anaerobic capacity. Only six sessions of continuous hills are done. This progression is repeated twice in the training year. The goal of the workout is to run as many hills as possible in the allotted time.

WEEK 2	Theme: Work to work
Monday	1 × 10-minute run at 70 percent; 5-minute recovery; 3 × 5-minute runs at 75 percent; 3-minute recovery between runs
Tuesday	24 × 30/30 at 75 percent Strength training: total body Core strength
Wednesday	Active rest
Thursday	8 minutes of continuous hills; 3 minutes of recovery + 4 minutes of hills + 5 minutes of hard running Strength training: total body Core strength
Friday	45-second run, 60-second run, 75-second run, 60-second run, 45-second run at 80 percent effort; rest is the time of the next run
Saturday	30-minute steady run at 70 percent effort of game
Sunday	Rest

(continued)

Figure 7.3 *(continued)*

WEEK 3	Theme: Recover and go
Monday	1 × 10-minute run at 70 percent; 5-minute recovery; 3 × 5-minute runs at 75 percent; 3-minute recovery between runs
Tuesday	20 × 30/30 at 80 percent Strength training: total body Core strength
Wednesday	Active rest
Thursday	8 minutes of continuous hills; 3 minutes recovery + 6 minutes of hills + 5-minute hard run Strength training: legs Core strength
Friday	Agility: footwork and change of direction
Saturday	Field circuit #1 × 3 Core strength
Sunday	Rest

NOTE: For the core workout on Tuesday, the players are provided with a training handbook that has core modules detailed. They can choose whatever modules they want, but they cannot do the same module for two sessions in a row. Saturday's circuit is designed to develop strength endurance. It involves exercises combined with runs of various lengths between the exercises.

WEEK 4	Theme: More quality work
Monday	Speed acceleration Agility: footwork
Tuesday	Staircase 30/30s (30-second runs at various intensities): 70%-75%-80% x 2 sets (3-minute jog rest) 75%-80%-85% x 2 sets (3-minute jog rest) 80%-85%-90% x 2 sets (3-minute jog rest) Strength training: total body Core strength
Wednesday	Active rest
Thursday	Hill sprints 12 x 100 meters Strength training: legs Core strength
Friday	Agility: footwork and change of direction
Saturday	Field circuit #1 x 3 Core strength
Sunday	Rest

NOTE: Tuesday's staircase 30s is a mixed aerobic and anaerobic session. It is a very tough workout that fosters a transition to more gamelike training.

WEEK 5	Theme: Focused hard effort
Monday	Speed acceleration Agility: footwork
Tuesday	Staircase 30/30s Strength training: total body Core strength
Wednesday	Active rest
Thursday	Hill sprints 12 x 100 meters Strength training: legs Core strength
Friday	Agility: footwork and change of direction
Saturday	Field circuit #1 x 3 Core strength
Sunday	Rest

WEEK 6	Theme: Take it up a notch
Monday	6-minute run test (how many meters in 6 minutes)
Tuesday	Staircase 30/30s Strength training: total body Core strength
Wednesday	Active rest
Thursday	Hill sprints 10 x 100 meters Strength training: legs Core strength
Friday	300-yard shuttle test
Saturday	Field circuit #1 x 3 Core strength
Sunday	Rest

Collegiate off-season programs like this are always quite a challenge. Two concerns are how to monitor and gauge progress and how to ensure that the training is done correctly. The success of the season is dependent on this phase of training. Given the relatively short length of the collegiate season, if the players are not fit at the beginning of training, there is not enough time to get them significantly fit. The key is that all players know the program before they leave school and that they use the manual and follow the workouts. To ensure this, the workout must be simple, it must not demand much in terms of facilities or equipment, and it must be accomplished in a reasonable time frame.

DYNAMIC 3-D FLEXIBILITY

Even though flexibility is a key component of training, it is misunderstood, misapplied, overemphasized in certain instances, and underused in other circumstances. It falls under the broad umbrella of work capacity because it can be a limiting factor in effective performance of other training components. Limits in functional flexibility can significantly impair the ability to move efficiently. Flexibility is a good example of the application of the principle of context. In context, flexibility is very beneficial; taken out of context, it can be detrimental. Flexibility is closely related to strength and posture. Functional flexibility will create a dynamic three-dimensional active range of motion of body segments for the required motor task. Three-dimensional implies control around the joint in all three planes of motion. Flexibility is not an end in itself, and flexibility and stretching are not synonymous. Stretching with all its variations is a means of increasing flexibility.

Traditionally, flexibility is defined as range of motion around a joint. A more suitable definition is range of motion around a joint with control. The key is *control*. If the range of motion is uncontrolled, then there is hypermobility (extensive flexibility), which is undesirable. Increasing range of motion is fine as long as an athlete can control that range of motion. In most instances it is the athlete who is hypermobile; the athlete who has joint laxity (no control) has a real problem. There are no valid norms for flexibility; every person has unique muscle elasticity, ligament laxity, and body structure. Flexibility is also event and sport specific. Just like balance and posture, it is a dynamic, not a static, quality.

To better understand the role of flexibility in movement, it is helpful to think of it in terms of the concept of mostability. This is a term coined by physical therapist Gary Gray that is descriptive of the function of flexibility. Mostability is motion with stability. It is the correct amount of motion, at the correct joint, at the correct plane, at the correct time. Development of flexibility demands an eclectic approach by applying what has been used for years in martial arts, dance, yoga, tai chi, and physical therapy. The concept of mostability will guide the development and application of a functional flexibility program.

To further define a functional flexibility program, refer to the movement constants in chapter 2 and examine the effects of gravity and the ground on the body. There are muscles that chronically shorten because of their location in the body and the function they perform. These are muscles that need to lengthen through functional movements. They require constant attention in maintaining quality of movement and in preventing overuse. Normal daily activities and repetitive motion of a sport activity can lead to chronic shortening. The muscle groups that require constant attention in terms of lengthening are the gastrocnemius and soleus, psoas, hamstrings, adductors, iliotibial bands, latissimus dorsi, pectoralis, and wrist flexors. These should be addressed daily depending on the sport and individual needs.

Flexibility training must be tailored to meet the needs of each athlete. It is possible to have two athletes in the same event or position who have entirely different flexibility needs. A limit in range of motion can compromise technique or affect the ability to either accelerate or decelerate over a full range of motion. Flexibility has a direct role in performance of certain sports. "Qualitative flexibility is clearly important in sports such as gymnastics, diving, ice skating, and dance. Also flexibility might improve performance under specific conditions in other sports. At the same time, it is not clear whether there is a flexibility threshold for optimal performance or that additional flexibility in already flexible athletes is necessary or desirable" (Thacker et al. 2004, p. 375). Consider the flexibility requirement of the sport as part of the sport demands analysis, but be sure to consider the needs of the individual athlete. Seldom does a flexibility deficiency appear in isolation; it is usually related to a deficiency in strength and sometimes posture. The qualities of flexibility and strength are closely related. I have seen so-called tight athletes significantly improve flexibility by undertaking a balanced strength training program.

In terms of training, flexibility is considered a separate unit. It should be addressed daily. As with any other training component, variation must be programmed into the flexibility routines. Flexibility is not a warm-up! It is *part* of warm-up, not the major focus in the warm-up. As a separate training unit to address specific deficiencies, flexibility is best placed after the

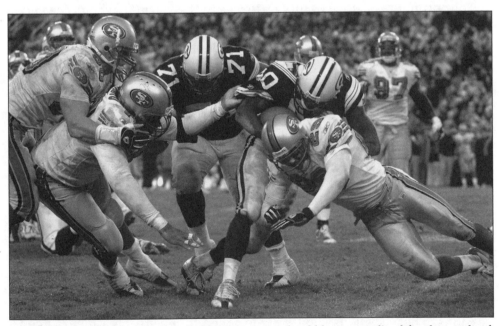

To achieve motion with stability, flexibility training should be personalized for the needs of individual athletes.

© Rob Tringali/SportsChrome

warm-up. The rule to remember is warm up to stretch, not stretch to warm up. Static stretching (that is, stretching that involves no motion) is best placed at the end of the workout as part of a cool-down because it restores the muscles to their resting length, which will reduce soreness and enhance recovery for the next workout.

Over the years the notion that preworkout static stretching can prevent injury has been continually reinforced. Numerous studies have shown little or no relationship between static stretching before exercise and performance or injury. Shrier (1999), in his extensive review of the literature, came to the conclusion that stretching before exercise does not reduce the risk of injury. After an extensive review of the studies pertaining to preexercise stretching and prevention of injuries, Thacker and colleagues (2004) also concluded that stretching was not associated with prevention of injuries. Despite this evidence, when an athlete pulls a hamstring or a groin muscle, the first assumption is that the athlete probably did not stretch enough. Some studies have shown static stretching to be harmful to performance. An unpublished study by Benton and Young (2001) on 10 national-level sprinters in Australia showed that when the group included static stretching before their starts from blocks, they were 3.38 percent slower than when they included dynamic stretching in the warm-up. The sample size was not large enough to show statistical significance, but a 3.38 percent difference in the performance world is significant to coaches and athletes.

For optimal results, flexibility exercises in the warm-up should be active (that is, involve movement) to facilitate the excitation of the nervous system to create a readiness for movement. The tempo of the stretches used in a warm-up is stretch, hold one count, relax, and repeat three times and then move on to another body part. The purpose of stretching in a warm-up is neural activation. Passive (involving the use of a partner or apparatus to hold the stretch) and static forms of stretching have a calming effect. That is appropriate for a cool-down or in a recovery session. It is inappropriate for a warm-up.

Deficiencies in range of motion can be remedied quite quickly, but sufficient work must be done to maintain those gains and to make sure those gains transfer to the activity. There are many tools to use for improving flexibility. The most adaptable tool is gravity. It is always available, easy to use, convenient, and effective. A balance point in the form of a rail, hurdle, or bench can enhance gravity. You can use towels or ropes to gain a lever advantage as an aid to stretching.

To improve flexibility, it is helpful to use a variety of methods. I have found it most effective to work on flexibility several times a day in shorter sessions. These sessions should be designed to meet each athlete's needs. Vary the duration of each stretch. For developmental stretching, hold the end position for 10 to 30 seconds. Some people advocate holding as long as a minute, but it appears that no appreciable gains are made after 30 seconds. Repeat the stretch three to five times. Dynamic range of motion is generally greater than static range of motion because tissue elasticity with dynamic range of motion is enhanced, leading to relaxation of opposing muscles during physical activity. The relevance of static flexibility to dynamic performance is an unresolved issue (Thacker et al. 2004). For this reason it is best to mix passive and active methods. In terms of progression, start active and then move to passive. Although not substantiated by research, experience has shown that stretching for 15 to 20 minutes approximately two hours after the final workout of the day is effective in reducing soreness and enhancing recovery as well as achieving noticeable gains in range of motion.

Two types of stretch receptors exist: one that detects the magnitude and speed of the stretch and one that detects magnitude only. Static stretches improve static flexibility and dynamic stretches improve dynamic flexibility; therefore, it makes no sense to use static stretches as a warm-up for dynamic action (Kurz 1994). This underscores the importance of carefully choosing the type of flexibility to be used relative to the type of workout.

The amount of work (time) required to maintain flexibility is significantly less than the amount of time required to develop it. Dynamic flexibility work is useful as an athlete's early-morning wake-up routine. Arm swings, leg swings, trunk rotations, reaches, and bending stimulate blood flow and wake up the nervous system. This type of stretching is a good foundation for further work during the day. With dynamic flexibility, athletes move parts of the body through progressively greater ranges of motion with gradually increasing speed. Movement should be flowing, rhythmic, and controlled. The repetition range is 8 to 12. Unfortunately, dynamic stretching is often confused with ballistic stretching. Dynamic stretching involves rhythmic swinging and rotation; ballistic stretching is done at maximum speed and offers no chance to change or correct the motion once it is started. Dynamic flexibility work will improve elasticity of muscles and ligaments.

Static stretches should follow dynamic stretches. Static stretching can be counterproductive if placed before a workout requiring explosiveness, speed, or agility. Immediately after static stretching the muscles are less responsive to stimulation, and coordination is thrown off. Static stretches interfere with the activity of tendon reflexes.

SUMMARY

Work capacity is the foundation of training. Paying attention to work capacity will allow athletes to train at a higher level and recover quickly from the work. Work capacity training enables athletes to work and compete at a higher level. It is more than developing an aerobic base; it involves developing an aerobic base relative to the sport. All components of work capacity are integrated in a complete training program. To avoid a negative effect on an athlete's training, flexibility must be addressed daily based on individual needs; other components do not need as frequent attention. Work capacity methods are threaded throughout the training plan in order to maintain work capacity. They are not developed and then forgotten.

Work capacity accumulates as athletes progress throughout a career. Therefore, it is not necessary to devote the same amount of time each year to development of the same capacities. The challenge as we move forward to discuss other components of athletic development is to maintain this work capacity base and not compromise the development of the other physical qualities. This is a delicate relationship that you must be constantly aware of.

Movement Aptitude and Balance

Effective athletic development is based on the development of fundamental movement skills before sport-specific skills. In generations past this was something that everyone took for granted because the demands of daily living took care of fundamental movement. People at all ages were much more active than they are today. Children grew up active, and free play was a major part of daily activity. It was natural to crawl, jump, hop, run, reach, lift, and throw; it was all done in a spontaneous, playful environment. Even in the adult world there were fewer conveniences than are available today. People walked instead of drove. Physical labor was part of daily life. People generally participated rather than watched. There was mandatory physical education from kindergarten through 12th grade in every state in the United States.

The athletic realm does not exist independent of the rest of society; athletes are a product of the society they grow up in. There is no longer mandatory physical education to provide a foundation of movement skills. There is less free play and more organized sport activity. The net effect of all this is a significant decline in fundamental movement skills. A sound athletic development program is founded on the basic locomotor skills developed to their highest level. These fundamental skills must be incorporated on a daily basis into athletes' training programs regardless of level of development. Obviously as athletes progress in training age and skill, fundamental skills should assume proportionally less of the training time. Ironically, in my work with high-level professional athletes I spend a good portion of training time on fundamental movements because they never acquired these skills as part of their foundation. Instead they specialized early and refined their sport-specific skills.

Fundamental movement skills fall into three broad categories: locomotor skills, stability skills, and manipulative skills (see figures 8.1 and 8.2). Locomotor skills are the skills that get us from place to place and cover the spectrum of the gait cycle from walking to running to sprinting. Swimming is also included in this category. Since humans are terrestrial beings, the emphasis in our athletic development program is on variations of gait. Stability skills are those movements executed with minimal or no movement of the base of support. Balance is a key element. It is a foundation of many sport skills, especially those involving finer motor patterns. A pitcher balancing on one leg to begin his delivery and a soccer player making a cut off of

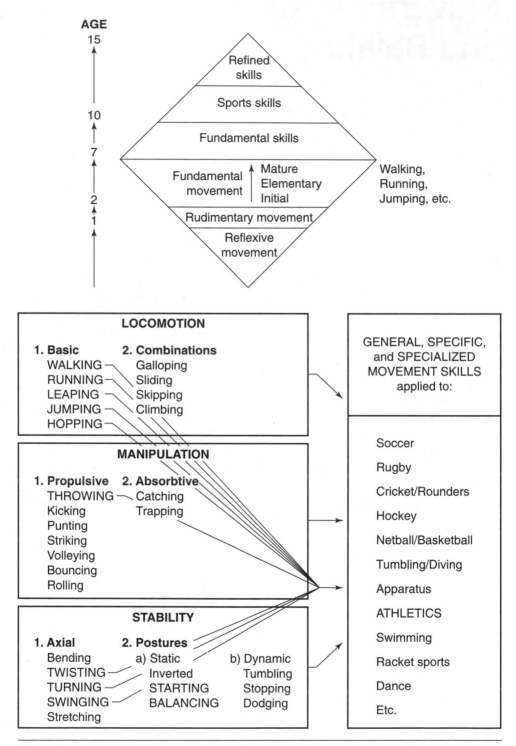

Figure 8.1 Development of movement abilities.

Adapted from C. Johnson, 1988, "Are we really going in the right direction?," *Athletics Coach* 22: 20.

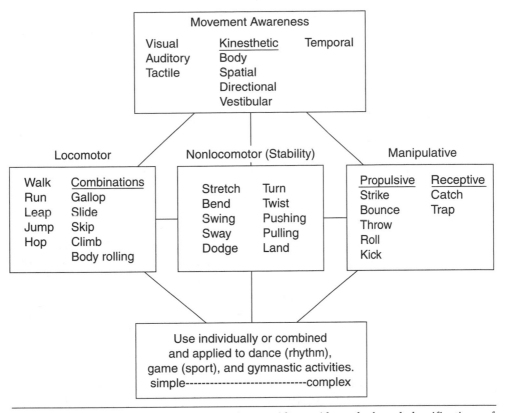

Figure 8.2   The basic movement categories provide a guide to the broad classifications of movement.

Fig. 2.7, p. 24 from PHYSICAL EDUCATION FOR CHILDREN by Clark Gabbard, Elizabeth LeBlanc and Susan Lowy. Copyright © 1987 by Prentice-Hall, Inc. Reprinted by permission of Pearson Education, Inc.

one leg are examples of this type of movement. Manipulative skills involve control of objects with the hands or the feet. Throwing and striking skills fall into this category. In our society the emphasis in manipulative skills is on work with the hands to the exclusion of the feet. This is a deficiency that must be addressed in an athletic development program. Better awareness and use of the lower extremities will pay rich dividends.

COMPONENTS OF MOVEMENT AWARENESS

To transfer (or translate) the broad movement categories into refined movement patterns, we need movement awareness. Movement awareness consists of those abilities necessary for conceptualizing and formulating an effective response to sensory information in order to perform a desired task or motor skill. This is *fund*amental work. It should be fun and mental in that it requires concentration. To train the components of movement awareness it is best to create an environment in which athletes are given a task orientation. This means that they are given movement problems to solve that will enable them to discover movement skills in a playlike environment.

A major goal of functional training is to incorporate movements that are part of sport skill movements so that they become automatic to the athlete. The best way to accomplish this is to have a nonawareness strategy. According to Ives and Shelley (2003, p. 180), "Nonawareness refers to a lack of attention placed on the activity while it is in progress, but learners are instructed to preplan the movement and focus on a specific situational cue." Nonawareness means having the athletes focus on solving a particular movement task rather than focusing on how they should move correctly. A good analogy is solving a word problem in math: You have to apply principles to solve the problem, and there may be more than one way to arrive at the solution. Movement is natural and instinctual; by making it conscious there is a high risk of making it robotic. Nonawareness allows for exploration and testing of limits to expand performance.

Most movement awareness activities can be addressed daily as part of a structured warm-up—structured in the sense that the thought and planning should be put into the sequence and timing of the activities, not the step-by-step orchestration or choreographing of the movement. The latter would defeat the purpose. Allow the athletes to express themselves. The goal is to create an environment where athletes can cultivate a rich repertoire of motor skills to draw on as a foundation for sport-specific skill. Proper form is highly individual. Relying on external means to stabilize a body part will not transfer to performance. The athletes get good at using the tool meant for correcting a movement error but they still do not get better at the task (Ives and Shelley 2003).

Crawling is one of the most important fundamental movement skills to emphasize in training, regardless of the level of the athlete. Crawling should be part of each day's workout. In more technologically advanced societies many children bypass the crawling stage or are not allowed to crawl because they are placed in various apparatus that limit their movement. This has dire consequences both in terms of motor and cognitive development. Crawling is the basis of reciprocal movement that underlies most sport skills. According to Hannaford (1995), "crawling, a cross-lateral movement, activates development of the corpus callosum (the nerve pathways between the two hemispheres of the cerebrum). The development of these pathways causes both sides of the body to work together to move the limbs, eyes, and ears. With equal stimulation, the senses more fully access the environment, and both sides of the body can move in a more integrated way for more efficient action." The closed-chain crawling position uses body weight to stimulate the scapular muscles with the abdominal wall and involves stability of the spine with cross-coordination when moving (McGrath 2001). There is no doubt that crawling must be part of every workout. The most logical place for crawling is in a warm-up, but it also can be part of a core workout (see chapter 9, The Critical Body Core). It wakes up many positive connections in the body.

A comprehensive functional athletic development program is built around the following components of movement awareness (Gabbard, Leblanc, and Lowy 1987):

• **Body awareness.** This consists of an awareness of all the parts of the body and their relationship to one another—the relationship of hips to feet (base of support) and hips to shoulders as well as eyes to hands and eyes to feet. A key to body awareness is awareness of center. Crucial to all movement and an integral part of body awareness is opposition. In gait it is the arms swinging in opposition to the legs. It is not something we should have to think about, but it is something we can train and take advantage of.

• **Spatial awareness.** This is awareness of the positions the body occupies in space. It is a sense of where you are in your environment. On the court or on the field it is sensing where you are in relation to the other people around you, even though they may not be in your direct sight. It is also a sense of where you are in tumbling skills and falling that allows you to control your body.

• **Rhythmic awareness.** Our fundamental rhythm is the heartbeat; all our bodily rhythms are derived from that. Sport movements are rhythmic in nature. This is highly related to music and dance. Movement is just a series of synchronous and asynchronous rhythms. To athletes it is a feeling, almost like an internal metronome.

• **Directional awareness.** This has two components: laterality and directionality. Laterality is awareness of both sides of the body, including how the sides work together and move to the side. Directionality is a sense of where you are going: forward, back, right, left, up, and down. The ability to move in all directions is a prerequisite for effective skill development.

• **Vestibular awareness.** This is the information based on feedback from the vestibular apparatus located in the inner ear that provides information about the body's relationship to gravity. It is closely related to balance and body awareness. The vestibular sense provides two key inputs: the position of the head in relation to the ground and the direction of movement in space. Mabel Todd (1937, p. 28) summarizes the physiology quite well: "the otoliths and semicircular canals are the seat of impressions of position and direction of motion in space; and they are combined in the brain with the kinesthetic sensations of movement, weight pressure, and relative position, coming from other parts of the body, to give us our minute-to-minute information as to the movements of our limbs, neck and trunk, where we are at any given moment, and how we can get somewhere else." This demands constant attention to head position and eye focus to guide the system.

- **Visual awareness.** Vision is a dominant factor in motor skill. Some experts have estimated that as much as 80 percent of all information we perceive is derived from visual feedback. Vision is closely tied to spatial awareness. It is the sense that modulates or regulates the other senses. This is a quality that is very trainable. It is also a quality that, if taken away by simply closing the eyes, can be used to heighten awareness of body position and balance.

- **Temporal awareness.** This is a sense of timing. This awareness is crucial for performance involving time constraints or a sense of pace. Temporal awareness is related to rhythmic awareness in terms of heightening awareness of the body's internal clock. It is an internal mechanism that can be trained.

- **Auditory awareness.** This is the ability to discriminate, interpret, and associate auditory stimuli. For smooth, efficient movement, auditory awareness must be highly developed. Hearing allows us to get feedback on the rhythm of movements. Something as simple as the sound of a foot strike in running is tremendous feedback to both the coach and the athlete.

- **Tactile awareness.** This is the sense of feel and touch. There is a tendency to think of this as involving only the hands, but feel and touch with the feet are also very important. The whole body is a giant sensory organ, so try to get away from thinking of tactile awareness as the exclusive domain of the hands. This component comes into play in a sport such as football, where the interior defensive lineman must feel the pressure of the block. Combative sports such as judo and aikido demand heightened tactile awareness in order to feel the opponent.

Ultimately, what links all the components of movement awareness into a complete functional program is proprioception. Proprioception is awareness of joint position derived from feedback in the sense receptors in the joints, ligaments, tendons, and muscles. It is a highly trainable quality. It is almost too simple. Coaches must strive to constantly change proprioceptive demand throughout the training program. In fact, this variable should be manipulated more frequently than exercise mode because it adapts so rapidly.

As you learned in the discussion of the performance paradigm, proprioception gives the quality to the motion derived from the interplay of force reductions and force production. Awareness of motion, weight, and position of the body originates within the body. This awareness is derived from reaction to gravity, inertia, and momentum. According to Mabel Todd (1937, p. 27), a dance professor concerned with precision and quality of movement, "Altogether, the proprioceptive system, acting in conjunction with all the other senses, serves to guide our total reaction to the outside world in terms of motion toward or away from particular objects, and to give us our ideas of space and time. More than any other factor the proprioceptive system is responsible for the appearance of the individual as an organized unit when he is moving about." Proprioception is the guidance system, essentially a gyroscope that puts the body and parts of the body in position to execute a skill. Proprioception is highly trainable. As far as incorporating it into training, I like to think of it as background music. It is always there. Coaches always must be aware of creating a proprioceptively enriched and challenging environment with the primary goal to enhance the quality of movement. This can be significantly enhanced if it is trained in the context of an appropriate cognitive environment.

POSTURE

In terms of execution of all the previously mentioned motor skills, posture is a vital component in the process. Dynamic postural alignment and subsequent dynamic muscle balance are the basis for all training. Posture is a dynamic quality; it is not static. It is not a still position posed in front of a posture grid. Posture is highly individual to each person's body structure and highly adapted to the sport activity an athlete is engaged in. According to Logan and McKinney (1970, p. 149), "The mature athlete tends to have a posture which is related to his particular sport if he has trained for years to become expert at his specific position or event. The reason for this phenomenon is the fact that the body tends to adjust or adapt to the various stresses or demands imposed upon it as a result of prolonged muscular activity." A good example of this is Lance Armstrong, six-time Tour de France winner, who evolved a position on the bike that is not considered perfect. Some experts were considering changing his position on the bike. The team chiropractor's answer to them was, "It's an imbalance, yes, but it's also Lance Armstrong" (Coyle 2005, p. 50).

Posture is a dynamic controlling quality. It is helpful to think of athletic movement not as one posture but as a series of postures. Optimal dynamic alignment of the segments of the kinetic chain yields coordinated movement. If one segment, or link, in the kinetic chain is out of sync, it sets up the potential for performance errors as well as a predisposition to injury if the movement is repeated often enough. The antigravity muscles of the core play an important role in maintenance of posture; they give the body structural integrity to allow the limbs to position and reposition according to the demands of the activity. Therefore, these muscles must be given prime consideration in a conditioning program. As mentioned in chapter 2, gravity is essentially trying to smash your body into the ground when you are just standing still. Add the complexity of running, jumping, or throwing, and it is easy to see how important antigravity muscles are in determining successful postures for performance. The body is fundamentally asymmetric. It is unrealistic to think of muscular balance as right to left or front to back. We must think of proportionality and get away from the idea of ideal posture; we must think in terms of individual needs and adaptations.

Posture allows the body to maintain normal relationships between length and tension in the muscles. Each posture in movement is a momentary alignment of body segments. Successful movement is determined by the ease of movement into the next posture. Much of the visual imagery in athletic movements is derived from still photos of static positions. This reinforces the mistaken notion of posture as a still position. Therefore, when you assess posture and subsequently train posture, it should be in motion, not in stillness. Static posture has very little relationship to movement unless there is some evident pathology or deformity. Once athletes begin to move, especially in a chosen skill pattern, everything seems to smooth out and even up. Also, posture is highly dependent on strength, flexibility, balance, and fundamental movement skills. Any deficiencies will result in compensations. Sometimes athletes can succeed in spite of the compensations, but invariably deficiencies have a way of coming back to haunt athletes. A sound strength training program coupled with an individualized flexibility routine can go a long way toward correcting any postural deviations that could interfere with efficient movement.

BALANCE

Balance is another component of athletic development that is highly trainable. Balance is essentially control of the center of gravity over the base of support. It is a dynamic quality, highly dependent on the blending of neural and physical components. It is also dependent on vestibular awareness. Balance can be subdivided into static and dynamic balance. Static balance is the ability to maintain equilibrium when the body is stationary. An example is balancing on one foot. Dynamic balance is the ability to maintain and control posture while moving.

Movement is a state of dynamic equilibrium involving a constant interplay of imbalance and balance in order to perform efficient movement. Balance is the ability to reduce force at the correct time, at the correct joint, in the correct plane, in the correct direction, for the required activity. There is a continuous reaction to gravity and external forces, such as the playing surface and opponents' actions. Maintaining this state of dynamic equilibrium requires systemic involvement with feedback from the ocular, vestibular, kinesthetic, and auditory senses.

It is convenient to visualize, test, and train balance statically. But as with posture, there is often very little carryover from static balance to dynamic movement. Therefore, when assessing balance, look at it as a dynamic quality. That is not to say that static balance should never be tested and trained. In training and assessment, static balance is the starting point in a progressive approach to balance training. Balance is significant enough as a performance factor that it should be incorporated into each workout. But it should be incorporated as a component when working on other qualities.

Remind yourself and your athletes that movements are essentially balance in motion.

Balance is involved in all athletic activities. For example, in sprinting, where at the world-class level the sprinter is on one leg for less than a tenth of a second at a time, it is a high-demand balance activity. In many sport activities it is highly task specific and trainable; therefore, it will be threaded through many workouts. Since most human motion is reciprocal in nature, in which movement shifts from one limb to the other (alternates), balance is a key mechanism in the execution of these activities.

To train balance it is essential to keep expanding the balance threshold, which is the distance you can move outside the

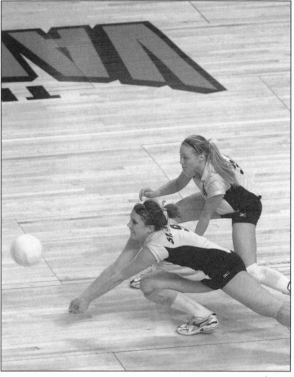

Training dynamic balance requires improving athletes' abilities to react to external forces and move outside their base of support.

base of support without losing control of your center of gravity. It is the point where balance is lost. Once it is lost it is not regained. For training purposes it is helpful to think of the body as surrounded by two cylinders. One cylinder is the inner-zone balance with all the parts of the body inside the base of support. The second cylinder, considerably bigger, allows the body parts to extend out beyond the base of support until the balance threshold is reached. Inner-zone balance work tends to be more static; outer-zone balance work involves reaches, steps, and full movements, so it is much more dynamic.

Athletes need to be aware of and effectively use the drivers of balance. The drivers are who or what is controlling balance. Essentially it is anything that manipulates the force a person has to balance against. In broad categories it is gravity, ground reaction force, or momentum. In most cases it is a combination of the three. Possible drivers of balance are an opponent or partner, gravity, angle of the ground, surface, shoes, direction of movement, arms and legs, and weight or stretch cord.

At this juncture a word of caution about balance training is warranted. It is not a matter of constantly introducing external drivers to make balance more difficult. Many experts today are advocating progressively more difficult unstable-surface and destabilizing products such as a balance board, foam rollers, and stability balls ad nauseam. That is not what balance training is about. Keep in mind why you are doing what you are doing—remember context. You are training athletes to improve performance in their chosen endeavor; you are not training for circus tricks. You will want the balance work to apply to the activities that athletes are training for.

Give much thought to a detailed progression. A simple progression begins with static balance and moves quickly to dynamic balance predicated on variations of the gait cycle. The last step is ballistic balance, in which the center of gravity is projected in large movements. Think of it this way: Stand, step, bound, hop, and then turn. Let your creativity and the sport demands analysis take you from there. The following are variables that you can manipulate or combine in a balance progression:

- Progress from bilateral (two-leg) to single-leg stance.
- Take the arms or the legs out of the movement as counterbalances to aid balance.
- Challenge vestibular demand by closing the eyes or moving the head; or if appropriate, use a blindfold.
- Vary the surface within reason.
- Use apparatus such as balance beams, balance boards, and BOSU balls. Do not get carried away with this.
- Be more dynamic.
- Increase the range of motion.
- Increase the speed.
- Add reaction.
- Add an external kinesthetic stimulus such as a push or a pull from a partner.

Be creative, but use common sense. The components of the following balance progression can be sequenced as a segment of a daily warm-up. This balance progression is a good lead-in for teaching correct landing in the plyometric teaching progression. The static single-leg squat balance routine is a good sequence for a cool-down. These exercises reinforce several important components of training. Also static and dynamic balance can be good active rest activities in a workout. They do not require any significant energy expenditure but do keep the nervous system tuned.

Balance Progression

❶ Static balance

Single-leg squat

Hold 10 seconds at each position.

Sagittal: The nonsupporting leg is bent at the knee and hip. The knee is pointed straight ahead at 12 o'clock (*a*).

Frontal: The nonsupporting leg is extended out to the side (*b*).

Transverse: The nonsupporting leg is bent at the knee and hip and rotated back so the knee is pointing to 4 o'clock (*c*).

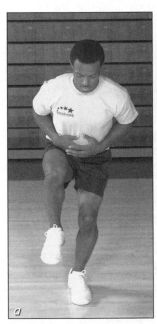 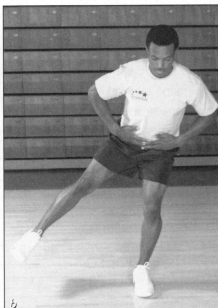 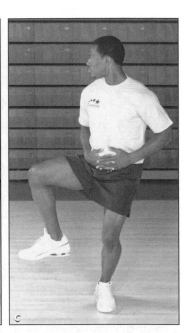

Do not progress to dynamic balance until the athlete can hold each position for 10 seconds with a minimum amount of sway. Also do not progress until the athlete can hold a low position on the squat.

❷ Dynamic balance

Hold 10 seconds at each position.

Sagittal: Step forward to balance on each foot.

Sagittal: Step backward to balance on each foot.

Frontal: Step to the side to balance on each foot.

Transverse: Step to 4 o'clock and balance on each foot.

❸ Ballistic balance

Bounds

Push off one foot and project out and up and land on the other foot. Stick and hold the landing as in a gymnastics landing. (Hold 10 seconds at each position.)

Sagittal: Bound forward to balance on each foot.

Frontal: Bound to the side to balance on each foot.

Sagittal: Bound backward to balance on each foot.

Transverse: Turn and bound to 4 o'clock and balance on each foot.

Hops

To hop, take off from one foot and project out and up and land on the same foot. Stick and hold the landing as in a gymnastics landing. (Hold 10 seconds at landing.)

Sagittal: Hop forward to balance on each foot.

Sagittal: Hop backward to balance on each foot.

Frontal: Hop toward the inside of each foot to balance.

Frontal: Hop toward the outside of each foot to balance.

Transverse: Turn and hop to 4 o'clock and balance on each foot.

❹ Balance training modules

It is best to do the exercises in this balance module barefoot to get maximum proprioceptive feedback.

Stepping stones

Use a combination of BOSU and 4-kilogram leather medicine balls. The balls should be placed a distance apart that challenges the athlete to reach and balance (*a* and *b*). Use 5 to 10 balls. Start with the balls in line.

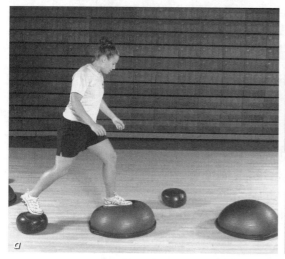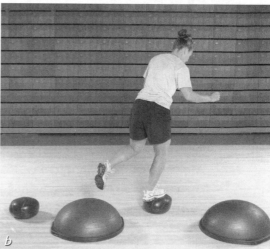

As the athlete gets more proficient, vary the pattern.

Step and close: Step onto the ball with one foot and then follow with the other foot so that both end up on the ball, then repeat to the next ball. Alternate leading legs.

Alternating-foot step, bend, and touch: This is the same movement as the previous exercise but bend and touch each ball with the hand opposite the leg that is on the ball. Do this at a controlled speed.

Single–double: Alternate stepping on one ball with one foot and the next ball with two.

Balance beam

The beam should be 8 feet (2.4 meters) long, 4 inches (10 centimeters) wide, and 4 inches high; it should lie flat on the ground.

Walk forward and back: Control the speed of the walk; do not rush.

Dip step: With each step, dip the nonsupporting foot below the beam.

Side shuffle: Maintain an athletic position throughout the movement. Step with the leading foot and follow with the other foot. Keep a shoulder-width base of support.

Single-leg squat: Squat by bending the ankle, knee, and hip. The speed of the squat should be as fast as possible while maintaining control and staying on the beam. Squat while positioned crosswise on the beam. Squat while positioned lengthwise on the beam.

SUMMARY

The training category of movement awareness can at first appear to be remedial. Just because it is remedial does not mean it is not important. All complex athletic skills are a succession of combinations of fundamental movements. Mastery of fundamental movements is crucial for athletic development and also for injury prevention. Some component of basic movement skill must be trained daily. Challenge athletes in this area, but don't make it a circus act. It should be sensible, and the athletes should feel the transfer.

The Critical Body Core

The core is a relatively new term in the lexicon of training. It is certainly a term that has taken on a life of its own. It is often used synonymously with *abdominals*, which is not completely accurate. The term *core* was coined by Bob Gajda and Robert Dominquez, two pioneers in the field of performance enhancement. They used the term in their seminal book *Total Body Training*.

The foundation of total-body training is the core, which comprises the muscles in the center of the body. These muscles stabilize the body while in an upright, antigravity position or while using the arms and legs to throw or kick. These muscles maintain the body's structure during vigorous exercises such as running, jumping, shoveling snow, and lifting weights overhead. These muscles also control the head, neck, ribs, spine, and pelvis (Dominquez and Gajda 1982). It is interesting to note that the term *core* did not originate in the lab with scientific research; it emerged out of practice and experience. Practitioners of martial arts have certainly understood the importance and function of the core for thousands of years. In martial arts it is called the *chi* or *ki*, the center of energy. In scientific terms it is the location of the center of gravity. Control of the center of gravity is essential for efficient movement.

It is helpful to visualize the core as a firm cylinder that surrounds the body and gives it structural integrity. The core muscles are involved in tonic (stabilizing) actions rather than phasic (movement). That means that the muscles function continuously while a person is moving, standing, or sitting (Dominquez and Gajda 1982). Core training improves dynamic postural control and develops appropriate muscular proportionality around the lumbo-pelvic-hip complex. A strong, stable core allows for the expression of dynamic functional strength and improves neuromuscular efficiency. Greater neuromuscular control and stability offer a biomechanically efficient position for optimal muscle function that leads to improved performance. Even though the core functions tonically to maintain stability, that stability is dynamic, ever changing. A strong core enables the body to assume various positions with instantaneous changes.

Understanding the serape effect is essential in understanding core function. This concept was articulated by Logan and McKinney more than 50 years ago. The serape is a Mexican garment that is draped loosely over the shoulders and is crossed in front of the body. The concept reinforces the muscles of the core as a connector. The serape muscles include the rhomboids, serratus anterior, external obliques, and internal obliques.

(See figure 9.1, *a* and *b*.) The serape effect involves several concepts that are vital to the understanding of movement. In ballistic actions such as throwing and kicking, the serape muscles involve internal forces. The muscles also transfer internal force from a large section of the body, the trunk, to smaller body parts, the limbs. In throwing, the serape muscles add to and transfer the internal forces generated in the legs and pelvis to the throwing arm (Logan and McKinney 1970).

The serape effect reinforces that in overhead activities there is a definite hip-to-shoulder relationship. According to Logan and McKinney (1970, p. 156), using the example of a right-handed thrower, "There is a definite interaction between the pelvic girdle on the left and the throwing limb on the right by way of concentric contraction of the left internal oblique, right external oblique, and serratus anterior on the right at the initiation of the throw. The pelvic girdle is rotating to the left and the rib cage is rotating to the right." This movement paradigm is true in all overhead activities. It is a rationale for training the core in diagonal and rotational patterns in order to take full advantage of core function. What is amazing is that there are still

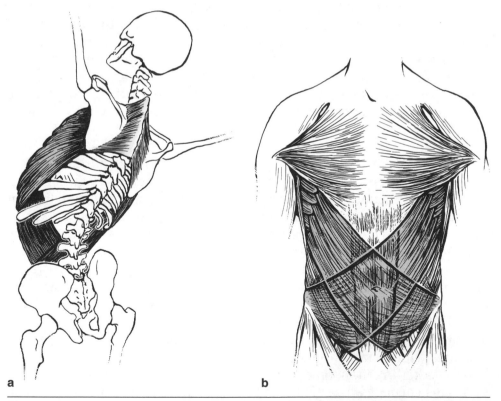

a   b

Figure 9.1 *(a)* The serape effect serves to reinforce the role of the core as a connector of the hip to the shoulder. *(b)* The muscles of the core work in diagonal rotational patterns based on their structure.

Reprinted from G. Logan and W. McKinney, 1970, *Kinesiology* (Wm. C. Brown Publisher), with permission of The McGraw-Hill Companies.

people who do not take advantage of this naturally occurring phenomenon. This has broad implications in performance enhancement as well as injury prevention and rehabilitation.

CORE FUNCTION AND TRAINING MYTHS

There are several myths and misconceptions about core function and training. One common myth is that there is an optimal firing order of the muscles and that this firing order can be consciously trained. The body is highly adaptable; therefore, it does what it has to do to move and protect itself. There is no optimal firing order. There may be firing order on the training table, but that does not transfer to a weight-bearing, gravity-enriched environment. The task that the core muscles must perform determines the firing sequence. In function the core muscles act as players in an orchestra: Each instrument (muscle) will have a different role depending on the music (movement) that is being played.

Another misconception arises regarding the role of individual muscles in core stability, specifically the transverse abdominis and the internal obliques. Many experts advocate consciously "drawing in" or "sucking in" the abdomen to recruit or isolate these muscles to provide core stability. Stability is not just a matter of activating a few targeted muscles. Sufficient stability is a "moving target" that continuously changes as a function of the three-dimensional torques required in supporting postures. It involves stiffening in order to sustain unexpected loads and preparing for moving quickly. Fitness in motor control is essential for stability and for avoiding injury (McGill 2002). Remember the principle of training movements, not muscles. No two isolated muscles can perform the function of stabilizing the trunk. As far as "drawing in," it is not something you need to consciously do. On exertion it is a reflex to exhale and tense up, which is known as bracing. Abdominal bracing makes the muscles stiff as opposed to hollowing the abdominal cavity, which is the result of drawing in. The act of hollowing does not ensure stability. Bracing activates the three layers of the abdominal wall; it is much more effective in enhancing stability of the spine. Hollowing is a classic example of misinterpreting scientific research studies and taking the results out of context.

The "six-pack abs" look is another misconception in core training. First, achieving the six-pack look requires significant reduction in body fat. Second, it requires an inordinate amount of work in one plane, the sagittal plane, to isolate those muscles. Essentially you would need to overdevelop those muscles, which have little role in functional movements. Athletes who move in many directions and have to control their limbs in a variety of positions have "ripped" abdominal muscles as a result of the movements they perform as opposed to isolated work. Good examples are jumpers in track and field and gymnasts. The demands of their sports produce strong, powerful abdominals as part of a fully functioning core.

Because the muscles of the core are always active, it only makes sense that we do not isolate those muscles. Work the muscles of the core in patterns that enhance motor control and coordination. All training is core training. When you lift overhead, squat, or bend, the core is active and working to dynamically stabilize and produce smooth, efficient movement. Without a fully functioning core, efficient movement is not possible. The body is a linked system, so functional core training is all about taking advantage of this linkage. It is about how all the parts of the chain work together to produce smooth, efficient patterns of movement. Remember, movement occurs from toenails to fingernails.

CORE MOVEMENT TRAINING

To truly understand core function in the context of function of the whole body, you must shift focus from muscles to movements. The brain does not recognize individual muscles. It recognizes patterns of movement, which consist of the individual muscles working in harmony to produce movement. According to McGill (2002, p. 144), "the muscular and motor control system must satisfy requirements to sustain postures, create movements, brace against sudden motion or unexpected forces, build pressure, and assist challenged breathing, all the while ensuring sufficient stability. Virtually all muscles play a role in ensuring stability, but the importance at any point in time is determined by the unique combination of the demands just listed." To enhance core function, you must carefully consider how the core will be activated in the activity you are preparing for. To train the core, train in positions that are similar to the movements in the sport activity you are training for. Think of patterns in which all the muscles of the core work together to produce smooth, efficient movement.

Gravity plays a huge role in core function. It is impossible to ignore gravity; it is essential for movement because it helps you to load the system. It dictates the postures that you will use to train the muscles of the core. If the sport takes place in a prone, supine, or seated position, then the majority of the core training should take place in those positions. If the activity takes place while standing, then the majority of the core training should happen while standing. The orientation of the body to gravity and its effects must be a prime consideration when designing and implementing a functional core training program, or you are not preparing the body for the forces that it must overcome and control.

The muscles of the core play a major role in the production and reduction of force, functioning as a big force transducer. There are 29 muscles that originate or insert on the pelvis; 20 of these link the pelvis to the femur, and the remainder link the pelvis to the spine. One of the best analogies is that the core is like the transmission of the car. Without a fully functioning transmission, the force that the engine produces cannot

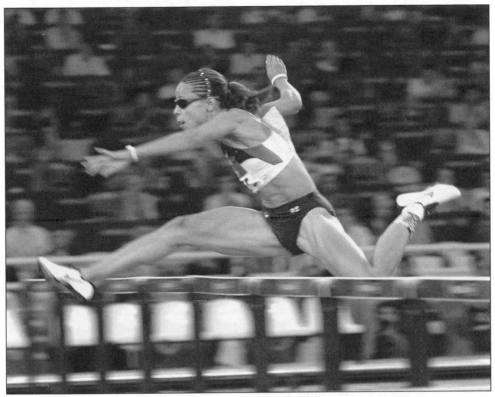

Core muscles that are developed through movement instead of isolation aid the production and reduction of force.

© Sport the Library

be transferred to the wheels. A good functional training program will work on the interplay between force production and force reduction with core training at the center of the program. Core training is the center of the training program because the core is trained daily and is active in all movements.

As discussed in chapter 8, posture is dynamic, not static. The muscles of the core play a decisive role in balance because of the location and function of the core muscles; therefore, core training and balance training feed off of each other. Training one will put demands on the other.

ASSESSMENT OF CORE STRENGTH

The ability to assess core strength is essential in order to design a specific core strengthening program. Traditionally assessment has been done with athletes in a prone or supine position with the goal of isolating relative strength of individual abdominal muscles. A functional assessment, on the other hand, involves integrated movement in a standing position or a position that simulates the posture of the sports as well as the gravitational demands.

For functional assessment, do the following: Perform a qualitative analysis consisting of a video of the athlete doing the respective sport activity from the front, side, and rear. Use the multiple views to judge quality of movement and assess any deficiencies that might stem from inability of the core to dynamically stabilize. The next part of the assessment consists of movements driven from the top down using the medicine ball, such as a chest pass for distance off two legs and off one leg. Compare the distance achieved from the throw off of two legs to the throw off of one leg. Also compare the distance achieved from the throw off the right to the throw off the left. Next do an overhead throw for distance off of two legs and off of one leg. Compare the distance achieved from the throw off of two legs to the throw off of one leg. Compare the distance achieved from the throw off the right to the throw off the left. Then a rotational throw is done. The athlete does the throw while facing away from the direction of the throw. Compare the distance of the throw with rotation right and left. To complete the core assessment, use tests that are driven from the bottom up. Use balance reach tests, lunge tests, and excursion tests or lunge, hop, and jump tests to complete the picture of core function.

Closely observe where successes and failures occur or where abnormal compensations occur. Is there any pain? If there is pain, what movement causes the pain? What movement is pain free? This method of assessing core strength takes into consideration the whole body. Relate these movements to any deficiencies in movement in the chosen sport.

PLANNING PROCESS FOR CORE TRAINING

Core training should be incorporated daily throughout the training year. Volume and intensity should be regulated in concert with the total workload and the objective of the particular training cycle. For power athletes, the emphasis should be on ballistic methods. For endurance athletes, the emphasis should be on stabilization methods. In rehabilitation of the upper extremity, stress the relationship between the core and the upper extremity. For the lower extremity, stress the relationship between the core and the lower extremity.

There are two principles of functional core training. The first is to train core strength before extremity strength. It is tempting and easy to do extensive work on the arms and the legs. But that will all be for naught if sufficient core strength is not developed first, because the limiting factor will be the lack of core strength. Therefore, in designing an effective program, always place core training first. This is true within a workout and also in a long-term plan. Dynamic postural alignment is the foundation for functional training. The key word here is *dynamic*—ever changing. The core controls dynamic posture, so the core will receive constant emphasis in the training programs.

The second principle is that all training is core training. This is because of the role that the core plays in all movements. Remember to integrate for function because the core works as an integrated functional unit that accelerates, decelerates, and dynamically stabilizes the body during movement. All movement is relayed through the core. The core functions as a swivel joint between the hips and the shoulders, which allows the entire body to accelerate, decelerate, and support the limbs.

Use the assessment to develop a core stabilization routine that is systematic, progressive, and functional, beginning with the most challenging position the athlete can control. Not everyone should start a program at the same place. Choose exercises that work the core in all planes of motion. Table 9.1 shows the distribution of exercises based on the movement classifications. The exercises should incorporate all of the following movements:

- Trunk flexion and extension (sagittal plane)
- Lateral flexion (frontal plane)
- Trunk rotation (transverse plane)
- Combinations (triplanar diagonal rotational patterns)
- Catching (triplanar diagonal rotational patterns)

The distribution of core training throughout the training year should be as follows:

- General preparation block: six sessions per microcycle
- Specific preparation block: four to six sessions per microcycle
- Peak competition block: three sessions per microcycle
- Transition block: two sessions per microcycle

Table 9.1 Distribution of Core Exercises

	Day 1	Day 2	Day 3	Day 4	Day 5	Day 6
Stabilization	Daily	Daily	Daily	Daily	Daily	Daily
Flexion and extension	Minor emphasis	Major emphasis		Minor emphasis	Major emphasis	
Rotation	Major emphasis	Minor emphasis	Minor emphasis	Major emphasis	Minor emphasis	Major emphasis
Throwing and catching		Major emphasis			Major emphasis	

To distribute the core work throughout the microcycle, you need to classify the exercises into broad movement categories. This will help to make the connection in understanding core function. The movement categories include the following:

- **Stabilization.** Basically all exercise involving the core will have a stabilization component.
- **Flexion and extension.** Exercises in the sagittal plane emphasize bending and extending.
- **Rotation.** Exercises in the transverse plan emphasize twisting.
- **Throwing and catching.** The very nature of throwing and catching will work the core through all three planes and demand dynamic stabilization.

Many core training tools are available. They all can be effective if used properly. Among the most common tools are body-weight (gravitational) loading, stability ball, body blade, power ball or kettlebell, dumbbell, stretch cord, medicine ball, wheel, and BOSU. Remember the adage "If the only tool you have is a hammer, then everything becomes a nail." Beware of overreliance on one tool. Remember the principle of variability. Use each tool individually. Learn the advantages and disadvantages of each tool. Combine tools with a specific purpose and goal in mind. Combine the tools with environmental modifiers in a sensible and logical progression. Constantly evaluate exercises and environmental modifiers relative to the continuum of function and the demands of the sport activity being trained.

Be sure to change only one variable at a time. The goal is a functional program, not confusion. You can manipulate the program by changing any of the following variables of program design:

- **Plane of motion.** You can design exercises to dominate in one plane, but for optimal core stability and transfer, it is probably best to use multiplanar movements.
- **Range of motion.** Limit range of motion only if absolutely necessary. Work through the fullest range of motion the athlete can control.
- **Loading parameters.** All of the following devices can be used exclusively or at times in combination: stability ball, dumbbell, tubing, weight vest, body blade, and medicine ball.
- **Amount of control.** Whatever the movement, there must be an element of control. If an athlete cannot control the movement, then the athlete should not be doing the movement.
- **Speed of execution.** This should be as fast as the athlete can control.
- **Amount of feedback**. The mode of exercise and the weight of the implement will provide feedback.
- **Duration.** This consists of the sets and reps of the actual exercises.

- **Frequency and density.** With core work it is beneficial to have some core training each day.
- **Posture.** This is perhaps the biggest transition in core training. The realization that the core is activated and must stabilize in a variety of positions and postures has opened up many possibilities. The chosen posture of exercise is determined by the posture of the sport. Core exercises performed while sitting and kneeling can limit rotation of the hips. Therefore, exercises in the sitting position will not be used except in sports such as kayaking, cycling, and possibly wrestling. The standing position has very strong application to most athletic movements. The lying posture (both prone and supine) is not as effective for integrating the muscles of the core as was once believed. Crawling, as discussed in chapter 8, is a very basic developmental phase of movement. It links the hips to the shoulders. Core work done while walking will activate many muscle synergies and carry over to specific sport movements.
- **Stance.** For throws and rotational movements the stance can have a big impact on the stress of the movement. A bilateral stance, involving standing on two legs with the feet shoulder-width apart, is also referred to as double support. A unilateral stance involves standing on one leg; it is also called single support. In the stagger, or stride, stance one foot is placed in front of the other to cause one side to dominate in a throwing or rotational movement. Solo refers to movements executed without a partner. Partner refers to movement executed in conjunction with another person.

There are many things to consider when selecting exercises. Safety is a prime consideration. To avoid the risk of injury, use only exercises that an athlete can control. The exercises must be sufficiently challenging to elicit an adaptive response. Stress multiple planes wherever possible and practical. Incorporate a multisensory environment without getting too extreme. All the movements should be derived from fundamental movement skills. The movements should be as sport specific as possible.

Progression is the cornerstone of the plan. It is potentially as harmful to artificially slow the movement down as it is to go too fast. Start with simple movement and gradually increase the complexity, but only as mastery of the simple movement is achieved. Start with familiar movements and then proceed to unknown movements. Progress from lower-force to higher-force movements and from static to dynamic movements. Maintain correct execution when increasing reps, sets, and intensity. Add external resistance where necessary. Increase proprioceptive demand through various forms of external loading only after previous steps in the progression have been mastered. The key to execution in terms of speed is to go as fast as an athlete can control. Always emphasize quality before quantity; never sacrifice the quality of the movement.

Because of the structure and function of the core, relatively high volumes are necessary for achieving any significant training adaptation. For rotational movement, the exercises are usually done in sets of 20 repetitions. For total-body throws, the rep range is usually 6 to 10. For wall throws or partner throws, the repetitions are 20. Select a maximum of 10 exercises in a session and base the number of reps on the training objective for each session. Allocate 15 to 20 minutes daily for core work. Rotations, chopping, flexion, and extension movements are especially effective as a warm-up. The throws should be done as a segment of the actual workout or as an actual workout to ensure high intensity and proper mechanics. Probably the least desirable time to train the core is after the workout or during a cool-down.

The following sample is a core training program for an overhead athlete. This program is appropriate for a baseball pitcher, football quarterback, tennis player, swimmer, javelin thrower, and fast bowler in cricket. The commonality in core function among this group of athletes is that the core functions to position and reposition the upper extremity in order to apply optimal force and then stabilize and reduce force during deceleration. Table 9.2, *a* to *c*, on pages 175 and 176 displays the distribution of work that should be used for different times of the year for the overhead athlete. Observe how the volume of work is distributed over each microcycle. The exercises do not change; rather, the sets and reps change. Therefore, athletes do not need to learn new routines when the cycles change.

Core Training Program for an Overhead Athlete

❶ Basic rotations

Walking wide twist × 20

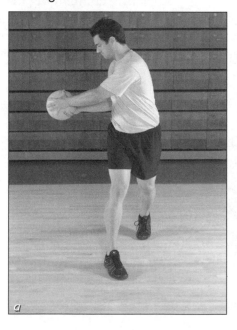
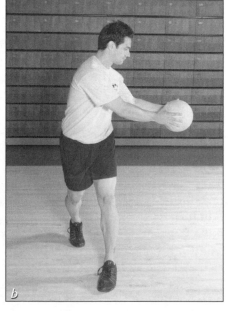

Walking tight twist × 20

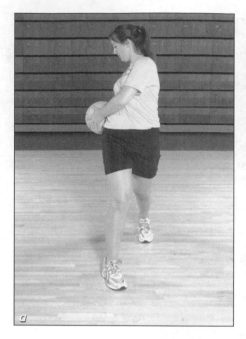 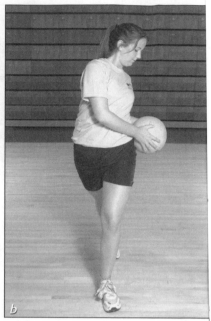

Walking over the top × 20

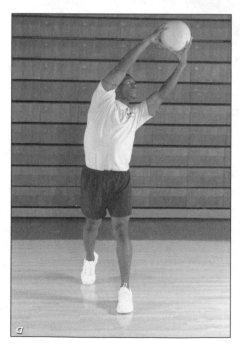 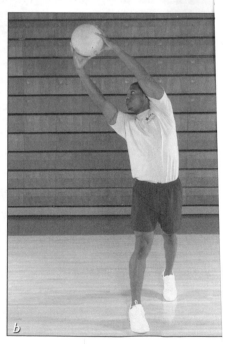

Walking figure eight × 20

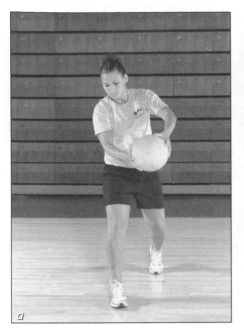 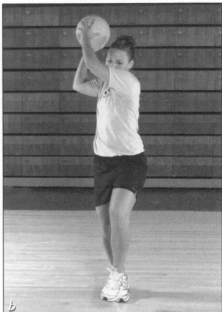

Base volume = 2 sets of 80 repetitions

These are performed each session as a warm-up.

➋ Core trainer (stretch cord)

Flexion and extension × 20

Twisting × 20 (10 each side)

Chop × 20 (10 each side)

Big circle × 20 (10 in each direction)

Base volume = 80 repetitions

Low volume = 2 sets of 80 repetitions

Medium volume = 3 sets of 80 repetitions

High volume = 4 sets of 80 repetitions

This can be done with a partner or solo with the stretch cord attached to a secure anchor point.

❸ Medicine-ball rotations

Standing full twist × 20 (10 each direction)

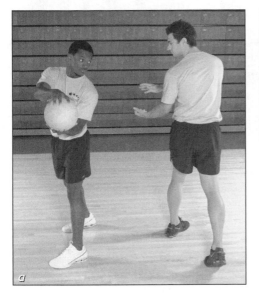 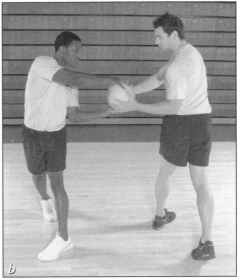

Standing half twist × 20 (10 each direction)

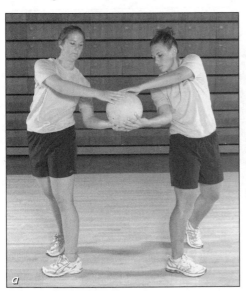 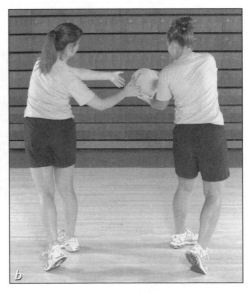

Half chop × 20 (10 each way)

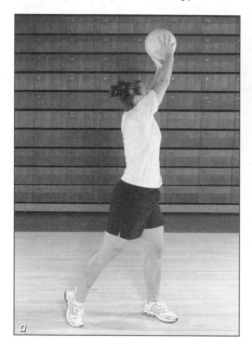 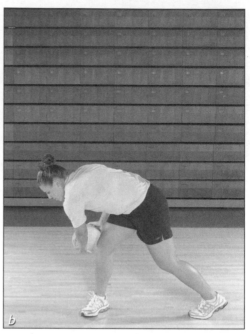

Seated V-sit throw × 20

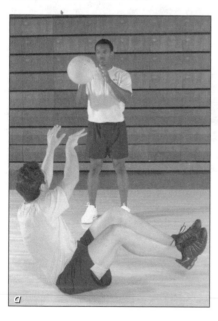 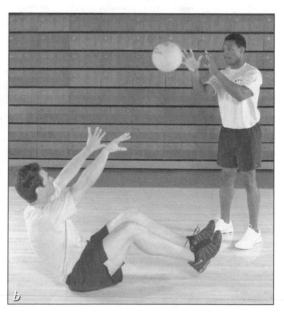

Seated side throw × 20 (10 each side)

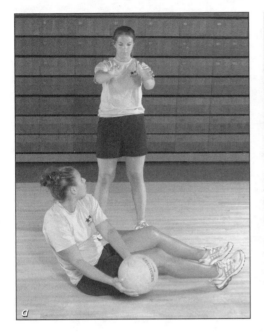 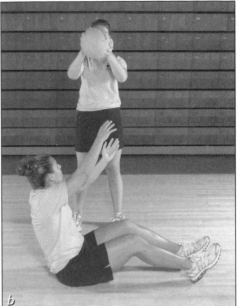

Solo medicine-ball sit-up (two positions right and left) × 5 reps each side

Base volume = 105 repetitions

Low volume = 2 sets of 105 repetitions

Medium volume = 3 sets of 105 repetitions

High volume = 4 sets of 105 repetitions

❹ Medicine-ball partner or wall throws

Overhead throw × 20

Soccer throw × 20

Chest pass × 20

Standing side to side × 20 (10 each side with cross in front)

Standing cross in front × 20 (10 each side)

Around the back × 20 (10 each side)

Base volume = 120 repetitions

Low volume = 1 set of 120 repetitions

Medium volume = 3 sets of 120 repetitions

High volume = 5 sets of 120 repetitions

❺ Medicine-ball total-body throws

Single-leg squat and throw × 12 (6 each leg)

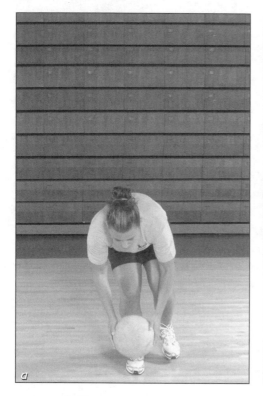

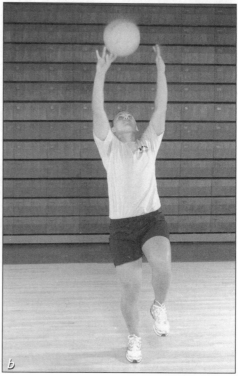

Single-leg squat and scoop throw × 12 (6 each leg)

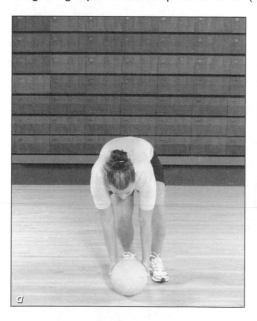

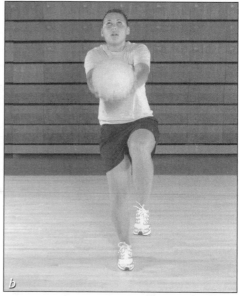

Over-the-back throw × 6

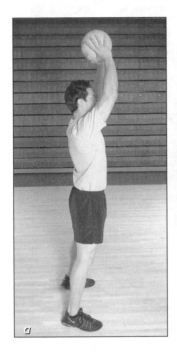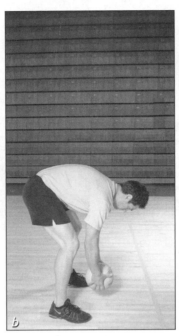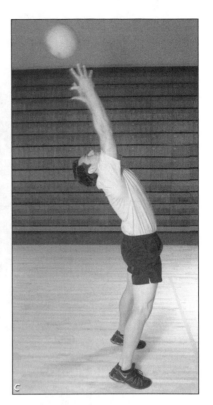

Forward through the legs × 6

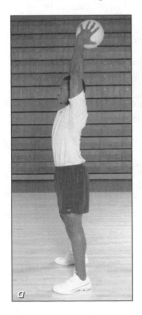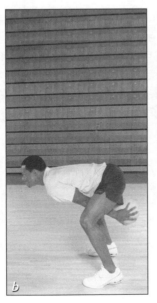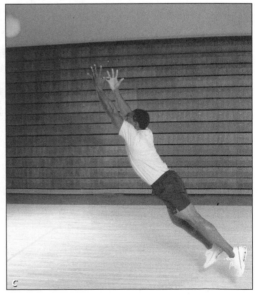

Squat and throw × 10

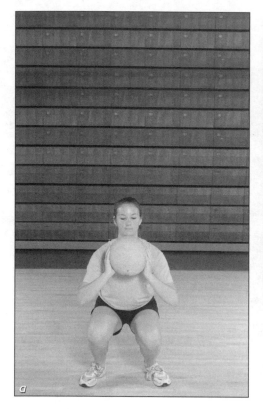 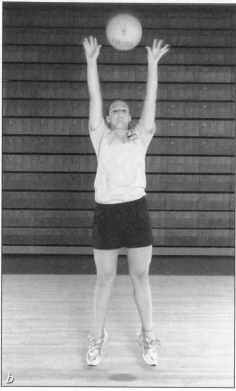

Base volume = 46 repetitions

Low volume = 1 set of 46 repetitions

Because these exercises are used to excite the nervous system and to achieve maximum explosiveness, they are never done for volume because fatigue would compromise explosiveness.

Core training program for an overhead athlete adapted, by permission, from Gambetta, V., and S. Odgers. 1991. *The Complete Guide to Medicine Ball Training*. Sarasota, FL: Optimum Sports Training.

Table 9.2a   Work Distribution for an Overhead Athlete in a Noncompetitive Cycle

	Day 1	Day 2	Day 3	Day 4	Day 5	Day 6
Basic rotations	Part of warm-up	Part of warm-up	Part of warm-up	Part of warm-up	Part of warm-up	Part of warm-up
Core trainer	Medium volume	Low volume	Low volume	Medium volume	Low volume	Low volume
Rotations		High volume		Low volume		Medium volume
Wall throws		High volume			Low volume	
Total-body throws	Low volume			Low volume		

Table 9.2b   Work Distribution for an Overhead Athlete in a Competitive Cycle

	Day 1	Day 2	Day 3	Day 4	Day 5	Day 6
Basic rotations	Part of warm-up	Part of warm-up	Part of warm-up	Part of warm-up	Part of warm-up	Part of warm-up
Core trainer	Low volume	Low volume	Low volume	Low volume	Low volume	Competition
Rotations		Low volume		High volume		
Wall throws		Medium volume			Low volume	
Total-body throws	Low volume		Low volume			

Table 9.2c   Work Distribution for an Overhead Athlete in a Peak Competitive Cycle

	Day 1	Day 2	Day 3	Day 4	Day 5	Day 6
Basic rotations	Part of warm-up	Part of warm-up	Part of warm-up	Part of warm-up	Part of warm-up	Part of warm-up
Core trainer	Low volume	Low volume		Medium volume		Competition
Rotations			High volume			
Wall throws		Medium volume				
Total-body throws	Low volume				Low volume	

SUMMARY

The concept of the core is relatively new to the lexicon of training. We must reinforce that the core is more than the abdominals; it comprises the whole torso. It is not about appearance; it is about function. Functional movements of the core will incorporate all three planes of motion, often in combination. This is necessary for training the core for the strength and stability required in athletic movements.

Because it plays such a prominent role in the center of the body, the core is a factor in all movement. And because the core is in the center of action in movement, it should occupy a central portion in training. Core training should be threaded through each session and through each training week to enhance the quality of movement and to prevent injury. A strong and functionally stable core will ensure superior movement with the highest efficiency. Never lose sight of the fact that all training is core training.

Full-Spectrum Strength

In the athletic development process, strength training is possibly the most important area because it is the underlying quality of so many other components. Strength and all its manifestations play a key role in posture. Strength is a prerequisite for speed and for jumping. It is a prominent factor in injury prevention. In the athletic development process, some thread of strength training is always present. At times, depending on the sport and the time of the training year, it will be highly visible and at other times it will be almost undetectable.

Traditionally strength training conjures up images of big muscles and heavy weights. That certainly can be part of it, but for the majority of athletic environments that is not the case. *Strength* is a term that incorporates a spectrum of activities and training methods, all of which are designed to meet the force requirements of the particular sport.

My experience with strength training spans over 40 years. I began weight training as an athlete in the early 1960s and incorporated strength training in my training programs when I started coaching in the late '60s. At that time the myths surrounding the negative effects of weight training were pervasive. The benefits and application to sport performance were not well established. Individual athletes and teams that made extensive use of systematic strength training programs were the exception rather than the norm. Track and field (athletics) and to a certain extent American football were the two sports that pioneered the application of strength training. It just so happened that those were the sports that I was involved in, so that exposed me to a variety of methods.

The functional path in strength training requires a significant departure from conventional wisdom. It is not about methods and modes of strength training; it is about the interaction of the body, gravity, and the ground. From sport science research and experience we now have a good grasp of the application, timing, and sequence of the various methods. Perhaps the biggest task today is separating scientific fact from marketing hype. The functional path is a multidimensional approach involving athletic movements designed to transfer into improved performance. The guide to the functional path is eclectic and practical. It involves a progressive spectrum of resistance modes culminating in high-speed, high-force activities. Strength training for athletic performance involves the application of basic concepts:

- Train movements, not muscles.
- Train core strength before extremity strength.

- Build strength from the bottom up.
- Incorporate pulling, pushing, and squatting movements that enhance linkage.
- Overload to force adaptation.
- Sensibly vary the mode and the load. Incorporate systematic planned variation, a key to strength acquisition and application.

There is no doubt that strength training should play a prominent role in the process of athletic development, but because of this it can become a trap. This occurs because, unlike many other physical qualities, strength gains are fairly rapid, measurable, and quantifiable—in the training setting as weight lifted or in the research setting as feet per pound (or centimeters per kilogram) of force expressed on a dynamometer. The role of strength training is to condition the bones, tendons, ligaments, and muscles to withstand and overcome the high forces placed on them in the demands of competition and training. It is easy to get sidetracked in the initial stages of strength training. When the window of adaptation is large, improvements in strength occur very rapidly. There is a linear relationship of work to improvement: The more you do, the better you get. It is only natural to assume that this will continue when, in fact, after the initial adaptations occur, it is necessary to change the stimulus. This is especially true with maximal strength training methods. Once a base level of maximal strength has been achieved, each time the athlete returns to that type of strength stimulus, he or she will not require a significant amount of time to return to previously acquired strength levels. Once those pathways or circuits are opened, it is easy to reopen them and tap into that strength reserve. The best approach seems to be to invest a significant amount of time initially for acquisition and then return to it for shorter, more concentrated periods designed to either tap into the reserve or to further stimulate growth. Of course, some of the distribution depends on the strength requirements of the sport. The football lineman and shot-putter will have more concentrated periods of maximal strength repeated more often than the tennis player or soccer player will. Virtually every sport needs some maximal strength training.

APPLICATIONS OF STRENGTH TRAINING

Strength training serves a multitude of functions depending on the sport and the athlete. A low-volume, high-intensity explosive lifting session will stimulate the nervous system before a high-quality sprinting session. The workout program designed to increase muscle mass will benefit football players and hurt soccer midfielders. A strength training program is a delicate balance that must fit within the context of the whole athletic development process. I know from experience how easy it is to let this get away from you. As an athlete I got caught up in the process and lost sight of the goal.

I spent too much time lifting and not enough time refining technique. As a coach I have stayed with cycles of strength training too long. The lesson that I have learned is that strength can be easily gained and easily maintained. It is maintained by doing a little bit more often. It does not require a huge time investment to maintain, just attention to detail and intensity.

Strength training is more than lifting weights. Perhaps the most important contribution of strength training is what is not measurable and visible. It is the constant work that must be done to develop and maintain strength in the synergistic and stabilizing muscles. Those muscles provide the framework for the muscles most involved in the various movements to reduce and produce force. The benefit of structural integrity in strength training has been overlooked. Some people call this stabilization strength; whatever you call it, it is the strength that lends quality to the movement. It is not measurable, but you sure can see it.

If you go back to the movement constants (chapter 2) as the basis of athletic development, you'll remember that gravity is one of the three movement constants. Strength training is gravity enhancement. As you add external resistance, regardless of the form of resistance, you are only enhancing the effect of gravity. Strength training assumes the degree of importance that it does because humans live, work, and play in a gravitationally enriched environment.

It is helpful to think of the concept of a weight room without walls. Because strength training is learning to cheat gravity and occasionally overcome it, you have so many more tools available for developing this quality outside the weight room. Not all strength training needs to take place in the weight room. As you look at the array of resistance methods available and the infinitesimal application of those modes and methods, this concept becomes very clear. At this juncture it is important to point out that this does not mean that it is not necessary to lift weights—quite the contrary. There is no question that the amount of time devoted to weight training is directly proportional to the amount of external resistance that must be overcome in the sport. It also relates to the collision or contact demands of the sport. If you must move an opponent or overcome the inertia of a heavy implement, then a significantly greater amount of time must be spent lifting heavier weights. If the sport is a collision sport, then there must be an investment in gaining muscle mass for protection. This has implications in exercise selection and program design, which are covered later in the chapter.

In athletic development, with the obvious exception of the preparation of a weightlifter or a powerlifter, strength training should be a means to an end. At times it will be the focal point of training and at other times it will play a subservient role. As we define strength and power and then move across the spectrum of strength training and detail the respective methods, be aware of where strength training fits. As athletes move through the spectrum, the goal is strength that the athletes can use, strength they can apply to their respective sports. It takes at least .6 of a second to generate maximum strength. Most sport performance takes place in less than .3 of a second. The main goal is to reconcile the difference. Sometimes this is very measurable in terms of weight lifted and number of reps; at other times it will manifest itself in less tangible ways. Developing applicable strength requires a vigilant approach so that the athletes and coaches do not get caught up in one method. It requires a thorough understanding of the demands of the sport from a perspective of strength and power, the pattern of injuries, and the qualities of the individual athlete.

COMPONENTS OF STRENGTH TRAINING

Strength is the ability to exert force. There are no time constraints—it is just how much force can be applied. Power, on the other hand, has a significant time element. It is the ability to express force in the shortest time. Think of power as the athletic expression of strength. Power flows; it is fast, explosive, and athletic.

Power can be broken down into speed-dominated and strength-dominated power. Strength-dominated power is characterized by the need to express high force against external resistance. Shot put, discus, and American football are activities that demand strength-dominated power. Speed-dominated power is characterized by restricted resistance. Throwing a baseball and swinging a golf club or a tennis racket characterize speed-dominated power.

One of the reasons that strength and all of its manifestations are so important is that it plays a role in all movements. In muscle action, strength will move a body part, it will resist movement of a body part, and it will stabilize (fixate) a body part. This all occurs within the context of a movement. Most of the traditional emphasis in strength training has been on the movement of a body part. Contemporary thinking has shifted so that strength training also needs to play a role in resisting movement of a body part, which is the eccentric component. Most injuries occur in the force-reduction phase. The role of strength in stabilizing a body part has been determined to be an important performance factor. A good strength development program will carefully direct training to address all three functions of muscle actions in an integrated manner.

There are several factors involved in gaining strength: neuromuscular, muscular, biochemical, structural, and biomechanical. All the factors should be taken into consideration in designing and implementing the optimal strength training program because they are highly interdependent. The neural component has probably gotten the least amount of attention because it is harder to "see."

Noted strength training researcher Dr. Digby Sale summed up the role of the nervous system: "Strength and power performance is determined not only by the quantity and quality of the involved muscle mass, but also by the extent to which the muscle mass may be activated by voluntary effort.

Further, the expression of voluntary strength and power may be likened to a skilled act, in which prime movers must be fully activated, synergists appropriately activated, and antagonists suitably inhibited. Strength and power training may cause changes within the nervous system that allow an individual to better coordinate the activation of muscle groups, thereby effecting a greater net force, even in the absence of adaptation within the muscles themselves. The possible changes within the nervous system that enhance strength and power performance may be referred to as neural adaptation" (Jones 1986).

The muscles are slaves of the brain. Ultimately it is the neural component that drives the system and enables the muscles to work. The nervous system, in response to the specific task, governs recruitment order. The brain does not recognize individual muscles; rather it recognizes patterns of movement. So the neural component provides a foundation of strength training: Train movements, not muscles.

The initial adaptation that occurs in strength training is neural. (See figure 10.1.) The body learns to engage the appropriate stabilizers and more effectively reduce and produce force. The neural adaptations manifest as

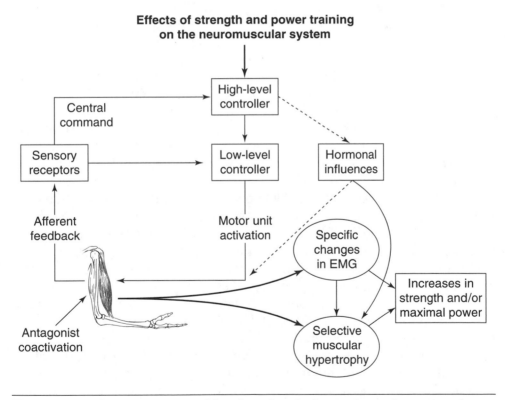

Figure 10.1 Schematic overview of the adaptations in the neuromuscular systems that occur with strength training.

Reprinted, by permission, from K. Hakkinen, 2002, Training-specific characteristics of neuromuscular performance. In *Strength training for sports*, edited by W. Kraemer and K. Hakkinen (Oxford, UK: Blackwell Publishing), 20.

increased firing rates and motor unit recruitment and improved motor unit synchronization. That is why when a beginner starts a program the initial gains are quite dramatic without any appreciable gains in hypertrophy (muscle bulk).

Maximum strength, also called absolute strength, is the highest force that can be exerted during a single voluntary muscular contraction. We know from practice and research that once those neural pathways have been opened, it is easy to go back and tap into those pathways. The analogy is that absolute strength is like a path worn across a grass field. As the path is traveled by more people, it is worn deeper and deeper. If the path is not used for some time, then the grass grows back. As soon as people start to walk on the path again, it is not long before the path is back. Absolute strength is much like the path. The lesson here is that once the maximal strength base has been established, you do not have to go back each training year and repeat the same loading cycles. Those cycles can be shorter and more intense to reopen the pathways. The other implication is that, based on sport demands, somewhere in the athletic development process maximal strength must be emphasized after a period of preparation for the heavy loading.

The limiting factor in both the acquisition and expression of strength is not the strength of the large muscles most involved (MMI) but rather the smaller stabilizing and synergistic muscles that guide and allow the expression of the strength development process. Functional strength is the ability to dynamically reduce and produce force through full range of motion with speed and control. It is a major contributing factor in smooth, coordinated athletic movement. It is not as measurable, but it is observable. An athlete with a high degree of functional strength may not be able to outlift everyone in the weight room, but the athlete can move, explode, and perform in the athletic arena with optimal efficiency.

Strength endurance is the ability to perform strength-oriented actions in a repetitive manner in a climate of fatigue. Once base-level strength has been developed, then it is possible to work on developing strength endurance. The traditional approach has been to start a strength training program with a cycle devoted to strength endurance. This is precisely how I was taught and what I did for the first years that I coached. I was never comfortable with this approach because, very simply, I thought the athletes were trying to endure a quality they did not have. If you don't have a base level of strength, how can you endure it? From this I derived the principle of strength before strength endurance. Therefore, in a sequence of training, the initial block will be devoted to acquisition of basic strength. Much of this is neural, or actually learning the movements. That allows athletes to lift more or perform more reps on body-weight exercises. Once that is achieved, then it is possible to progress to a strength endurance block.

CIRCUIT TRAINING

The primary means of developing strength endurance is circuit training. Circuit training is essentially interval strength training. A strength exercise is performed for reps or time. A certain rest interval is given and the athlete progresses to the next exercise. Circuit training is certainly not new; it simply has been rediscovered. The method of circuit training was systematized in England in the 1950s. It was used extensively in physical education curricula and in military training. For some reason circuit training fell out of favor. It is a method that I have continued to use over the years with great effectiveness, not just with sports and athletes in which the strength endurance demand is high but with speed and power athletes as a primary means of raising work capacity and changing body composition.

The obvious goal of circuit training is to develop muscular endurance, which has the added benefit of improving work capacity. In a team setting it is a very viable method because large numbers of athletes can train at one time. Circuit training also can be easily adapted to target specific areas of the body (such as the legs, core, or upper body) or address specific deficiencies. In setting up a circuit training program, carefully consider the following:

- You need to tailor the circuit to meet individual needs and rate of improvement.
- The exercises you select must be strenuous; exercises for the small muscle groups are not appropriate.
- The exercises need to be simple, since skill will break down as athletes fatigue.
- Standardize each exercise so that athletes can measure progress regardless of the circuit criteria.
- Recognize any bias in the circuit.

The actual circuit can be constructed in several different ways. Perhaps the most common and simple form of circuit training is a rep-based circuit in which an athlete performs a set number of reps of a particular exercise and then moves on to the next exercise. It is also possible to construct a time-based circuit. The time-based circuit is set up so that the exercises are performed for a certain amount of time with a fixed rest interval. The loads and exercises have to be carefully chosen so that athletes can work for the entire time prescribed. Progress is judged by the number of repetitions achieved. A combination of the two can also be used. For example, a good measure is to take total time for a rep-based circuit to measure progress.

I have not limited the use of circuit training to the preparation period of training, nor have I limited its use to the sports that had obvious strength endurance demands. It is a training method that can significantly improve work capacity and bring about significant changes in body composition. The key is to understand sport demands and individual strengths and weaknesses and then design specific circuits that can be used throughout the training year as a tool to enhance work capacity and serve as a good routine breaker. There is no question that circuit training is a demanding form of training. Because it is so demanding, it must be used judiciously. The longest that a block of circuit training should last is four weeks. Generally I will devote one block a year exclusively to circuit training and then thread circuit work throughout other blocks as a tool to stabilize work capacity. The following are some examples of circuits.

Core Circuit

In the core circuit, athletes do the prescribed reps at each station and move to the next station with no rest between exercises. This allows significant time under tension to develop core strength. In a core circuit without rest between exercises, six exercises would be the maximum number of exercises that can be used without compromising the quality of execution. If you feel the need to do more, then add multiple circuits of the same exercises with sufficient rest between circuits to ensure good execution.

1. Landmine rotation × 20 (10 each side)
2. Two-position sit-up × 20 (10 each side)
3. Stability-ball kickback × 20
4. Big circle × 10 each direction
5. Ab roller × 10

General Circuit

This is an example of an overall general conditioning circuit. Each strength exercise is performed for the maximum number of reps possible in the 30-second exercise period. There is a 10-second transition to allow the athlete to get the jump rope and then 30 seconds of jump rope. One or two times though the circuit is a very good workout. This is an especially good circuit to use with sports such as basketball or soccer in the first third of the competitive season, especially the day after a game.

1. Push-up and jump rope
2. Body-weight squat and jump rope
3. Kettlebell big swing and jump rope
4. Body-weight lunge and jump rope
5. Medicine-ball chest pass and jump rope
6. Combo I (curl and press) and jump rope

7. Medicine-ball big circle and jump rope

8. Body-weight lateral lunge and jump rope

9. Step-up and jump rope

10. Lateral step-up and jump rope

Leg Circuit

The leg circuit is the foundation for more specific strength work to follow in terms of absolute strength and plyometrics. This is a program I have used for years to establish a base of strength and power endurance. It is also a good tool to use in lower-extremity injury rehabilitation to rebuild a work capacity base in preparation for return to play. The basic requirement for progressing to heavier lifting and high-level plyometrics is the ability to perform five full leg circuits without stopping. When athletes have progressed to this point, they are ready.

1. Body-weight squat: 20 reps

2. Lunge: 10 reps each leg

3. Step-up: 10 reps each leg

4. Squat jump: 10 reps

The key to the effectiveness of the circuit is the speed of the repetition. The goal is one rep per second. This is not possible on the lunge and squat jump, but with those exercises it should be as close as possible to that rate. The squat should break parallel. The length of the lunge should be as long as the athlete is tall. The step-up is an alternating step up on a low box (14 inches or about 36 centimeters) high. On the squat jump the arms are held at the waist to accentuate the work of the legs. (See figure 10.2.) The leg circuit progression is twice a week on Monday and Thursday or Tuesday and Saturday. In terms of progression, the eventual goal is to go through the circuit continuously without a rest.

This circuit is very demanding. For an athlete who does not have a good training base, use the following progression. Do not take any shortcuts in the progression; it is very methodical and designed to produce results over the long term. Athletes need to execute the exercises with speed and full range of motion. The fast eccentric nature of the work will result in significant soreness, which is another reason to proceed methodically through the progression.

Leg Circuit for an Athlete Without a Good Training Base

Week 1: 3 circuits with 30 seconds between exercises and 1 minute between circuits

• Body-weight squat: 10 reps

• Lunge: 5 reps each leg

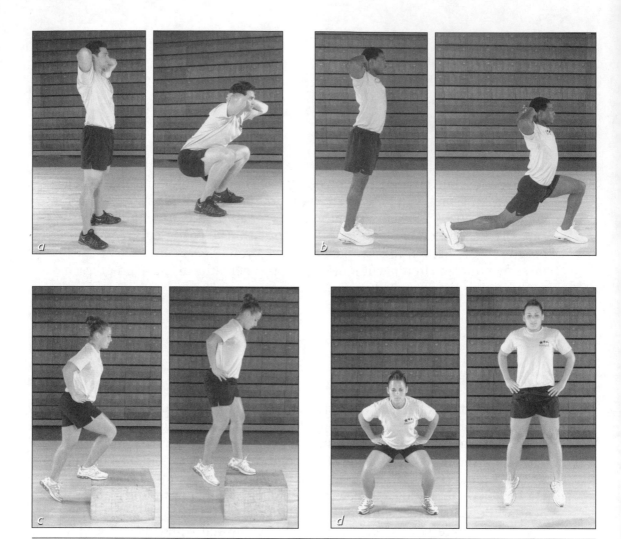

Figure 10.2 *(a)* Body-weight squat, *(b)* lunge, *(c)* step-up, and *(d)* squat jump.

- Step-up: 5 reps each leg
- Squat jump: 5 reps

Week 2: 5 circuits with 30 seconds between exercises and 1 minute between circuits

- Body-weight squat: 10 reps
- Lunge: 5 reps each leg
- Step-up: 5 reps each leg
- Squat jump: 5 reps

Week 3: 3 circuits with no rest between exercises and 1 minute between circuits

- Body-weight squat: 10 reps
- Lunge: 5 reps each leg
- Step-up: 5 reps each leg
- Squat jump: 5 reps

Week 4: 5 circuits with no rest between exercises and 1 minute between circuits

- Body-weight squat: 10 reps
- Lunge: 5 reps each leg
- Step-up: 5 reps each leg
- Squat jump: 5 reps

Week 5: Session 1—5 circuits with 30 seconds between exercises and 1 minute between circuits

Session 2—5 circuits with no rest between exercises and 1 minute between circuits

- Body-weight squat: 15 reps
- Lunge: 8 reps each leg
- Step-up: 8 reps each leg
- Squat jump: 8 reps

Week 6: Session 1—5 circuits with 30 seconds between exercises and 1 minute between circuits

Session 2—5 circuits with no rest between exercises and 1 minute between circuits

- Body-weight squat: 20 reps
- Lunge: 10 reps each leg
- Step-up: 10 reps each leg
- Squat jump: 10 reps

For athletes with a good base of training, use the following six-week progression. The exercise order is the same but the reps for each exercise do not vary. The reps are 20 for the squat, lunge, and step-up and 10 for the squat jump. The only things that vary are the sets and the rest between exercises and circuits. The total volume in reps for each workout is in parentheses.

Leg Circuit for an Athlete With a Good Training Base

Week 1: 3 circuits with 45 seconds between exercises and 3 minutes between circuits (210)

Week 2: 4 circuits with 45 seconds between exercises and 2 minutes between circuits (280)

Week 3: 5 circuits with 30 seconds between exercises and 90 seconds between circuits (350)

Week 4: 5 circuits with 30 seconds between exercises and 60 seconds between circuits (350)

Week 5: 5 circuits with 30 seconds between exercises and no rest between circuits (350)

Week 6: 5 circuits with no rest between exercises or between circuits (350)

STRENGTH TRAINING TRANSFER

There is no doubt that strength training for athletic performance has been heavily influenced by bodybuilding methods and heavy overload training from American football. These types of training, though very appropriate in the context they were designed for, do not always translate well to sports where muscle bulk and absolute strength are not necessary. Most sports require a high level of functional strength—strength that can be used. Functional strength training is strength training with a purpose.

The concept of transfer specificity is unclear to many coaches and trainers. Except for practicing the specific task or sport itself, no conditioning activity has 100 percent carryover. However, some activities have a higher percentage of carryover than others because of similarities in neuromuscular recruitment patterns, energy systems, and biomechanical characteristics. Yet most of the time, an athlete cannot use the sport or activity to gain the necessary overload on the neuromuscular system, and this is why resistance training is used in the conditioning process. This is why weight training has had such a dramatic effect on performance in the throws in track and field. Prior to resistance training, all the throwers did was throw the implement at competition weight. There was little overload in terms of external resistance. It is less about specificity and more about preparation for more specific work. In the quest to be "functional," perhaps we may become too concerned with making strength very specific to the sport and to the movements of the sport. Ian King, Australian strength coach, offers the following thought-provoking perspective (2000, p. 125): "I am more concerned about what strength training effects will transfer to sport performance than I am about specificity. In brief, I believe strength is general rather than specific, and attempts to make it overly specific risk losing many benefits of strength training."

Some coaches think that athletes just need to get stronger and address only the strength aspect of muscular performance; they also think that the movements of the sport will address the power component. This is a flawed premise because an athlete needs to train the characteristics of muscle that have the greatest effect on performance, and 1RM (one-repetition maximum) strength is only one of several trainable variables (such as power, rate of force production, local muscular endurance) in muscular performance. That is the rationale behind the spectrum approach that I advocate. The spectrum approach encompasses training all types of muscle action from slow-speed, high-force to high-speed, high-force ballistic movements. Each of these variables is unique and interacts to produce different training effects over time. Objectively evaluate each athlete's current strength and power levels relative to the strength demands of the sport, position, or event. What are the athlete's limitations? What type of strength does the athlete need? How much time does the athlete have?

The traditional approach to strength training is to prescribe workouts by sets, reps, and load. As an athlete progresses in training age, this approach can be too general and inconsistent in the results. In order for the strength training to transfer effectively to performance, a more accurate quantification of the quality of movement is required. You need to look closer at the speed of the bar and the actual force production in order to ensure transfer to performance. It is possible for two athletes to perform the same number of reps with the same weight and have very different effects. For example, if one athlete takes twice as long to perform the reps as the other athlete, then the power production is affected. Traditional systems have been based either on 1RM tests or on projected max calculated from the rep maximums. Technology is now easily available for obtaining a measure of bar speed and the resultant force. Start by measuring peak force in either a separate testing session or at the start of each training session. I prefer the latter because it is a more accurate reflection of an athlete's status on that particular day. From the measure of peak force, set the system at a certain threshold, such as 90 percent of peak force. Instead of performing a prescribed number of reps, athletes perform as many reps as possible until they can no longer produce the desired percentage of peak force. This ensures high-quality reps and high-force production. It is very motivating for athletes because more feedback is supplied from this method than from the amount of weight lifted. They quickly learn that peak force is higher when their technique is better. This changes the focus from just getting the bar up to attaining high-quality movement at speed.

OLYMPIC-STYLE WEIGHTLIFTING

In the athletic development process the role of Olympic-style weight training has assumed a large emphasis. This has good and bad implications. Olympic-style weightlifting is an excellent training method for developing power. It consists of two movements, the clean and jerk and the snatch. The derivatives of those movements are what make up the majority of the training exercises. There is no question of the inherent value of these exercises as a tool in raising explosive power, but once again the method must be kept in context and reconciled with the overall goal of the strength training program.

To achieve optimal return, you must consider several key points. The first point is that Olympic lifting is a sport. That sport consists of lifting as much weight as possible in the clean and jerk and the snatch. Those lifts have a high technical demand, but the skill is a closed skill that occurs in a narrow range of motion. The Olympic lifting movements do produce tremendous power because of the distance the weight must travel, the weight, and the speed requirements. This power production is highly dependent on the technical proficiency of the individual lifter. The training of the weightlifter consists of the actual Olympic lifts and some derivative and assistance exercises. There is no running, jumping, or other demands on the system.

Olympic lifters traditionally have lifted several times a day. This began in the 1980s because of the influence of the Bulgarians who emerged as a dominant power in the 1970s. The Bulgarian weightlifters were reported to have had as many as six lifting sessions in a training day, repeated for up to six training days in a microcycle. Each session seldom exceeded 60 minutes. All sessions were at very high intensity. Again, the point must be made that all these athletes did was lift. Also keep in mind that they were full-time "professional" athletes. Perhaps the most important underlying factor that enabled them to accomplish this severe training regimen was a program of systematic doping. We know that was a huge factor in the lifters' ability to recover and handle the high volumes of high-intensity work necessary for making the type of strength gains these lifters were making. Also keep in mind that on the international scene, Olympic weightlifting is the "dirtiest" sport in terms of positive drug tests.

The reason for pointing all this out is not to be negative or to denigrate the sport; rather it is to put the emphasis on Olympic lifting in perspective. Too many coaches have blindly copied the methods of the Olympic lifters without taking these things into consideration. Even if you are an Olympic lifting coach, the volumes and intensities reported from the Eastern bloc countries are beyond anything a drug-free athlete can possibly handle for any significant time. Richard Lansky, coach of Team Florida weightlifting, has found that a realistic adjustment in volume and intensity is in the range of one third less for his athletes than those commonly reported in Eastern European weightlifting literature.

Let's take this a step further. It has become very popular among the strength coaching community, especially in American football, to center strength training programs on Olympic lifting. Many of the football strength coaches blindly copied the volumes and intensities of the Bulgarian and Soviet lifters without taking into account the previously mentioned facts. This volume and intensity was applied in addition to the running, agility work, jumping, and sport-specific training. It should be easy to see the problems that would arise.

As mentioned earlier, the Olympic lifts are very technical in their demands. Typically athletes' lifting sessions are sequenced after their other work. This is not optimal time to use lifts with a significant technical element and high neural demand, because fatigue will compromise technique.

The other factor that must be considered when extrapolating from the world of Olympic weightlifting is body proportions. Olympic lifters, in effect, are preselected by their body types. To be successful, tall athletes with long limbs are quickly weeded out. Smaller athletes with shorter limbs (which afford a lever advantage) succeed. Therefore, applying Olympic lifting movements without taking into consideration body proportions can severely compromise the effectiveness of the methods. I have seen back injuries occur in tall basketball players who were required to perform various Olympic lifting movements without modifying the movements for their body proportions.

Another argument given for the use of the Olympic lifting movements is that they help with jumping because in biomechanical analysis of Olympic lifting, the pattern of force closely resembles the vertical jump. I may be missing something here, but then why not just jump with resistance? Learning and mastering the technical complexity of the Olympic lifting movements to improve jumping seem to be a stretch. In most situations when working with athletes, there is not an infinite amount of time available for training. Therefore, I choose methods that allow me to train athletes to be better at their sport within the constraints of the available time.

After all this, would I recommend using the Olympic lifting movements? Absolutely. I advocate their use for all sports because of their potential for power development, but you must adapt and modify the movements to fit each athlete—literally. Carefully consider body proportions. Make significant modifications for tall athletes. Note that the Olympic lifting movements do not have to be done with a bar. I have found Olympic movements with dumbbells to be particularly effective. The factor of body proportions is eliminated because the dumbbell will always "fit" the body. The disadvantage of the dumbbell is that an athlete will eventually be limited in the amount of weight that he or she can lift. So that if you are working with sports that require strength-dominated power, such as football or throwing, then the athletes will need to use the bar to achieve heavier loading. Dumbbells also allow modification of the pulling movements to be done in diagonal and rotational patterns. The bar essentially locks a lifter into the sagittal plane. Another interesting modification of Olympic lifting movements is the use of sandbags (see figure 10.3). This method has reportedly been used extensively by Jan Zelezney, world-record holder in the javelin. Sandbags not only allow an athlete to work in multiple planes, but they can be thrown, which significantly raises power production.

From a technical perspective, make sure that you as a coach know and understand the technique. Master the teaching progressions. Be sure to allow time in the training program for skill acquisition before adding significant loading. Also teach and preferably train the movements in a nonfatigued

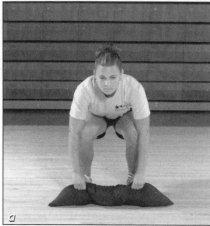

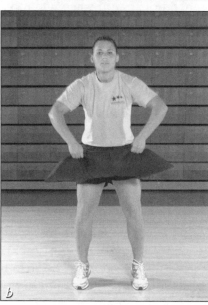

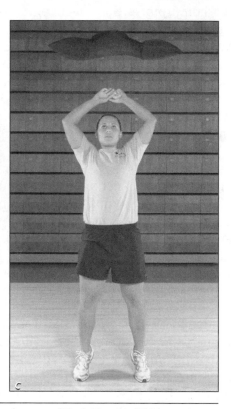

state. Adapt the method to the athlete; don't adapt the athlete to the method. Remember you are not training Olympic lifters; you are training athletes who use the Olympic lifts and derivatives to raise explosive power.

Figure 10.3 Sandbags can be used to perform modified Olympic lifting movements such as the snatch throw.

FREE WEIGHTS AND MACHINES

There seems to be an ongoing debate about the relative merit of free weights versus machines. In many circles this can be quite an emotional argument. Much of the emotion arises because of commercial considerations. In our consumer-oriented, high-tech society, the equipment manufacturers have inundated us with claims for the benefits of their line of machines. The high-tech appeal comes from the fact that machines look "high tech" and they can be made high tech by adding dials, digital readouts, and auditory beeps.

If you can objectively look at most machines from the perspective of the principles of functional sport training discussed in this book, there is not much of an argument about whether free weights or machines are preferable. Perhaps the biggest argument in favor of machines is that they are safe because the resistance is guided—you cannot drop the weight or accelerate it beyond the set range of motion. In reality, machines can be quite unsafe because the machine locks the body in; in fact, many machines provide Velcro straps to ensure that. Machines are designed for the average person, not the person who falls outside the norm. Therefore, the range of adjustment of the seats and lever arms is limited, which can cause the forces to be abnormally transmitted. Everything is fine if the axis of rotation can line up exactly with the center of the joint, but because of design and the varied body proportions, this is a difficult proposition.

Another disadvantage of using machines is that the athlete is seated in many of the machines. Most sport movements do not occur in this position. The body will not learn to effectively position and reposition its orientation to gravity if all the strength training is done in this environment. Even with machines done in standing positions, the resistance is guided, which allows a person to lean on the machine for stability. That allows someone to lift more weight, but it is an artificial environment that does not effectively transfer to unsupported movements.

Most machines allow movement in only one plane, primarily the sagittal plane. As already discussed, function demands movement in all three planes. Most machines isolate (that is, they work one joint). This definitely gives a burn, particularly when training to failure on that particular machine. From the perspective of functionally training an athlete, this is not an advantage. I am not interested in having an athlete feel the burn; I am interested in strengthening the movement, not the muscle, to better prepare the athlete for the forces that occur in the competitive arena.

Because most machines work one joint in one plane, athletes who train primarily on machines do get bigger. Isolating muscle groups and training slowly increase time under tension, which will stimulate growth. My concern is whether bigger truly is better. This type of lifting compromises overall athleticism in order to increase muscle mass.

Some machines can be very functional. Various rowing machines can be very useful in overloading the big muscles of the back. Some free-standing cable machines allow the point of resistance to be varied, which allows an athlete to train in a variety of positions in multiple planes involving multiple joints. Those are good machines to use, but if you did not have them you could still effectively train without them. As a coach I never want my athletes to be dependent on a machine or a device to train. I want them to be independent, to learn to tune in to their bodies so that the training can more effectively transfer to the competitive arena.

I do use several machines in training, but my strength training is never centered on those machines. If the machines were taken away, they could easily be replaced with a free-weight or a body-weight exercise. Evaluating machines from a standpoint of efficiency is also important. Only one athlete can be on a machine at any one time. Also, working the whole body requires several machines, which take up a lot of space.

In summary, it is not an argument of machines versus free weights; it is about understanding and applying the principle of training movements, not muscles. If the training tool, whatever it is, trains movements, then use it!

STRENGTH TRAINING PROGRAM DESIGN

Now you can put the theories and ideas into practice and look at the components of a sound strength training program. First of all, never lose sight of the ultimate product. What are the goals of the whole training program? Where does strength training fit in the spectrum of training methods that you can use in order to reach the ultimate objective? Frankly, that is where many strength training programs fail. They fail because they are not an integrated part of the whole program. There is one key to following the functional path: the principle of context. Keep strength in context.

A critical consideration in strength training program design is the correlation and interaction of the strength training with the overall training program. Seldom, if ever, will an athlete only strength train. Strength training must be carefully blended with the current overall training emphasis. Kraemer and Häkkinen (2002, p. 37) offer this advice: "The ability to better quantify the workout and evaluate the progress made toward a specific training goal is the hallmark of solid program design, which leads to optimal physical development. Resistance training programs have for many years been a source of mystery. Too often athletes just try to copy what the champion does, but this can be the formula for failure if the actual requirements of the athlete do not match the program used. Training goals are related to the specific types of adaptations needed, which in turn drive the performance outcomes. Thus, the best program is designed to meet the needs and goals of a specific athlete in the context of the sport."

Maximum power is the main determining factor for success in activities that require a sequence of movements leading up to release at high velocity or high impact at the end of the movement. To achieve maximum power production, an athlete must train both the force and velocity components of strength. There is a mistaken notion that to train the velocity component all that is necessary is to move the bar faster during a lift (Wilson et al. 1993). This has the opposite effect; it increases the deceleration phase because the athlete still has to stop the bar at the end of the lift. To achieve maximal power, the athlete must accelerate the bar or the implement throughout the entire movement. A major limitation of using weight training to achieve maximal power is that the bar must achieve zero velocity at the end of the concentric phase of the movement. This means that near the end of an exercise, whether it is a squat, clean, or bench press, the bar must slow down in preparation for stopping. Research has shown that in a maximal lift, 23 percent of the movement is accounted for by deceleration of the bar. In a lift at 81 percent of maximum, the deceleration phase accounts for 52 percent of the concentric movement (Wilson 1994). This can be overcome if the athlete jumps or releases the weight. What is the optimal load for achieving maximal power production? For the lower body the optimal load is 30 to 40 percent of 1RM. For the upper body the optimal load is 30 to 45 percent. Those percentages optimize force and velocity.

Maximal power training (MPT) exercises allow for the production of the highest forces possible throughout the whole range of motion. One of the best examples of this type of movement is the weighted squat jump. Multiple-repetition squat jumps are associated with power outputs usually generated only by elite weightlifters. During the second pull of the jerk thrust, multiple-repetition squat jumps may provide an excellent alternative or supplement to the traditional Olympic weightlifting movements for the development of speed strength. If space and time are limited, then the simplest method of raising maximum power production is the weighted squat jump (Baker 1995).

Throws with sandbags, weight plates, or other heavy objects raise explosive power. This type of work is effective in stimulating the nervous system during times of heavier sprint work where it would not be possible to do any extensive plyometric work. Maximum power training is at the high-speed, high-force end of the strength training spectrum.

Strength Training for Women

For female athletes the most important component of training for both performance enhancement and injury prevention is strength training. Of all training components, strength training can have the most profound effect on female athletes' improvement in sport. That does not mean that female athletes should *only* strength train; rather, strength training is a factor that should always be present in the training program regardless of the time of the training year or the stage in a career. Strength is not an isolated athletic quality; it has a profound effect on speed, suppleness, and stamina, not to mention skill.

Female athletes are usually deficient in strength for a myriad of reasons. Therefore there is room for improvement—a huge upside. There are no barriers. There is a tremendous ability to adapt to this stimulus with a positive spillover to all other components of athletic fitness. There is also an important positive psychological effect in terms of improvement in confidence and self-image. In regard to physiological differences, it is quite clear that the quality of females' muscle mass is quite trainable. No differences exist in the quality of muscle between males and females. The observed differences in absolute muscle strength are simply related to the quantity of muscle mass (McArdle, Katch, and Katch 2001).

Following are the physiological facts regarding strength training for females (Fleck and Kraemer 1997):

- **Muscle mass.** There is a difference in distribution of muscle mass. Women have less upper-body mass than men do. In the lower body there is less difference, but there's still a difference.
- **Absolute strength.** Obviously there is a fairly large difference between the sexes.
- **Relative strength.** Women are not as strong as men in the upper body, but in the lower body the difference is significantly less. When the strength is expressed relative to lean body mass, then the strength difference all but disappears.
- **Menstrual cycle.** Strength training has no more effect on the menstrual cycle than any other form of exercise.
- **Training effect.** The same adaptation and responses will occur in terms of strength acquisition in men and women.
- **Testosterone.** At rest men have 10 times as much testosterone as women, which has implications on the ultimate ability of female athletes to gain muscle mass.

The following are gains that female athletes can expect to achieve with a well-designed strength training program:

- There will be gains in lean mass if that is the objective, although the gains in mass are not as significant as they are in male athletes.
- The high-energy caloric density of the strength will cause a change in body composition (a loss of fat and a gain in lean mass).
- Female athletes are able to get a high return for the time invested; explosive power can be significantly increased.
- Muscular endurance will improve, which fosters performance improvement.
- The improved ability to handle body weight and control the body is crucial in the prevention of injuries, especially in the lower extremity.

Females mature earlier than males; therefore, girls should begin strength training earlier, preferably before puberty. It has been my observation (not supported by research) that female athletes who begin a well-rounded strength training program before puberty tend to be leaner after puberty. Females must strength train more often and continue throughout the competitive season because the drop-off in strength is more dramatic when strength training is stopped. Separate the boys and girls during the middle school years. There is too much difference in body composition between boys and girls, which can be discouraging to both boys and girls.

Strength Training Implementation

Ten specific steps compose the process of designing and implementing a functional strength training program. Follow the steps in the order presented to design the most effective program to meet the athletes' specific objectives.

1. Clearly define the goals of the strength training program. Be specific.

2. Ascertain how those specific goals fit in context with the total training program.

3. Select the exercises.

4. Classify the exercises in terms of general, special, or specific strength relative to the sport.

   • **General strength.** These exercises are directed toward the development of the force component of power. They are characterized by slower-speed, higher-force movements. Traditional weight training exercises and other resistance methods do not mimic any aspect of sport-specific skill. Speed of movement is of little or no concern. This is all about force, not speed.

   • **Special (transitional) strength.** The purpose of these exercises is to convert general strength into specific strength. These exercises could be considered similar but not the same as specific sport movements. Olympic-style weightlifting, medicine-ball work, stretch-cord work, and plyometric training usually fit into this category. A force component is present, but there is a higher speed component. The exercises are more specific than those for general strength.

   • **Specific strength.** These exercises are characterized by movement with resistance that imitates the joint action of the sport skill. There is a high degree of specificity in terms of mechanics, skill, and above all speed of movement. This obviously will have the highest degree of transfer to sport-specific skill.

5. Design the individual workouts.

6. Determine the order of exercises within the workout.

7. Classify the exercises as remedial, ancillary, or focus exercises.

   • **Remedial exercises.** These are basic strength training exercises designed to address basic movements. These exercises are designed to wake up the nervous system and work on the smaller synergistic and stabilizing muscles that often fail before the larger, more involved muscles fail. There is no need to have more than two remedial exercises in a daily program unless there is a specific deficiency that must be corrected. An example of a remedial exercise for the lower extremity is the single-leg squat. For the upper extremity an example is the push-up.

- **Ancillary exercises.** These are supportive exercises designed to prepare the body for the stress of the focus exercises. The movements are similar, and the load is usually less. The goal is to move in a stepwise progression to the heavier loading of the focus exercises. An example of an ancillary lower-extremity exercise is a front squat or even an overhead squat. For the upper extremity it is a dumbbell bench press or an alternating dumbbell bench press. There should be no more than three ancillary exercises in a workout or the exercises would detract from rather than enhance the focus exercise.

- **Focus exercises.** These exercises are the focal point of the workout. Traditionally these have been called core exercises, but that term is now associated with exercises for the torso. Everything in the workout is directed to these exercises. At most there should be two focus exercises in a session. The focus exercise is characterized by heavy-load and multijoint movement. Examples are the bench press and the squat.

8. Determine sets, reps, and intensity.
9. Execute the workout.
10. Keep accurate records and evaluate each workout in the context of the ultimate goal.

There is an obvious overlap between general, special, and specific strength. The amount of this overlap will vary with the athlete and the sport. In fact, a general exercise for one sport could be a special exercise for another sport. General strength will predominate during a general phase of training because it provides the base. Rather than think of the classifications as pure definitions, think of them as a continuum in which one classification overlaps the next classification.

Determine the cycles for strength training—once again, correlate this with the other training components. Distribute the exercises throughout the training week in one of two possible scenarios in order to net optimal return. In a four-day training week, distribute the work as follows: speed, power, recovery, strength, and work capacity. In a three-day training week, distribute the work as follows: speed and power, recovery, power and strength, recovery, and strength and work capacity. In both arrangements, the strength workouts are integrated with the other components to create a complete program.

SAMPLE STRENGTH TRAINING PROGRAM

I developed the following model over the past few years. It is an adaptable model that works very well in sports that do not require gains in muscle mass. It significantly raises power and work capacity and changes body composition. These phases must correlate with the technical workouts and the development of other global motor qualities. They must not detract from the quality of the other workouts. Intensity is the key throughout each phase. The workouts are not long, but they are very intense. They demand a high degree of concentration and attention to rest intervals and constant adjustment of load. The model must be adapted to each particular situation. I have found that most of the manipulation occurs in the length of the block relative to the competition schedule.

Foundational Strength

Emphasis: Total-body and multijoint movements with external resistance and body weight. See figure 10.4 on pages 202 and 203 for specific workouts.

Length of cycle: Four to six weeks.

Frequency: Four-day split.

Means: Stage training method. Total-body movements in a rep range of 4 to 6. Individual exercises with resistance in a rep range of 6 to 10. With body weight the rep range is 15 to 20 for upper body and 20 for lower body.

Basic Strength

Emphasis: Volume loading through push, pull, and squat sequence work. Figure 10.5 on pages 203 and 204 provides specific workouts.

Length of cycle: Four to six weeks.

Frequency: Four-day split routine.

Means: Stage training method. Dumbbell complex plus leg circuit, regular upper body.

Power Endurance

Emphasis: High-intensity work that is 20 to 30 seconds in duration with a 1:1 work-to-rest ratio in multiple sets. Emphasis is on total-body movements.

Length of cycle: Three to six weeks depending on the level of development of the athletes and how many times they have been through this model.

Frequency: Three days, on alternating days.

Means: Stage training method. Growth hormone work.

Table 10.1 provides an example of how I have implemented the power endurance phase into the training plan for a Division I university women's swimming team. This particular phase is sequenced as the third dryland training phase of the training year. This is the most intense and demanding of the dryland training blocks. There is competition during this phase, but all the competitions are developmental meets. The strength training emphasis here is based on the research that indicates that an intense 30-second work bout repeated with a 1:1 work-to-rest ratio for multiple sets significantly raises

Table 10.1　Power Endurance Phase for Division I Women's Swimming

Monday	Tuesday	Wednesday	Thursday	Friday
Week 1				
GH training: 3 cycles of :30/:30 1. Alternating high pull 2. High pull to press 3. Squat to press Legs: Squat 3 × 20 with weight	Incline push-up 2 × 15 Ring pull-up 2 × max Ring jackknife 2 × max Ring row 2 × max Dumbbell bench press 3 × 8 Dumbbell combo series: 3 cycles 1. Curl and press 6 2. Over the top 6 3. Wipe your nose 6 Parallel-arm step-up 3 × 20	GH training: 3 cycles of :30/:30 1. Alternating high pull 2. High pull to press 3. Squat to press Legs: Lunge 3 × 20 with weight	Incline push-up 2 × 15 Ring pull-up 4 × 15 Dumbbell bench press 3 × 6 heavy weight Ring row 4 × 15 Ring French curl 4 × 15 Dumbbell combo series: 3 cycles 1. Curl and press 6 2. Over the top 6 3. Wipe your nose 6 Parallel-arm step-up 3 × 20	GH training: 3 cycles of :30/:30 1. Alternating high pull 2. High pull to press 3. Squat to press Legs: Step-up 3 × 20 with weight
Week 2				
GH training: 4 cycles of :30/:30 1. Alternating high pull 2. High pull to press 3. Squat to press Legs: Squat 4 × 20 with weight	Incline push-up 2 × 15 Ring pull-up 2 × max Ring jackknife 2 × max Ring row 2 × max Dumbbell bench press 3 × 8 Dumbbell combo series: 3 cycles 1. Curl and press 6 2. Over the top 6 3. Wipe your nose 6 Parallel-arm step-up 3 × 20	GH training: 4 cycles of :30/:30 1. Alternating high pull 2. High pull to press 3. Squat to press Legs: Lunge 4 × 20 with weight	Incline push-up 2 × 15 Ring pull-up 4 × 15 Dumbbell bench press 3 × 6 heavy weight Ring row 4 × 15 Ring French curl 4 × 15 Dumbbell combo series: 3 cycles 1. Curl and press 6 2. Over the top 6 3. Wipe your nose 6 Parallel-arm step-up 3 × 20	GH training: 4 cycles of :30/:30 1. Alternating high pull 2. High pull to press 3. Squat to press Legs: Step-up 4 × 20 with weight

Monday	Tuesday	Wednesday	Thursday	Friday
		Week 3		
GH training: 5 cycles of :30/:30 1. Alternating high pull 2. High pull to press 3. Squat to press Legs: Squat 5 × 20 with weight	Incline push-up 2 × 15 Ring pull-up 2 × max Ring jackknife 2 × max Ring row 2 × max Dumbbell bench press 3 × 8 Dumbbell combo series: 3 cycles 1. Curl and press 6 2. Over the top 6 3. Wipe your nose 6 Parallel-arm step-up 3 × 20	GH training: 5 cycles of :30/:30 1. Alternating high pull 2. High pull to press 3. Squat to press Legs: Lunge 5 × 20 with weight	Incline push-up 2 × 15 Ring pull-up 4 × 15 Dumbbell bench press 3 × 6 heavy weight Ring row 4 × 15 Ring French curl 4 × 15 Dumbbell combo series: 3 cycles 1. Curl and press 6 2. Over the top 6 3. Wipe your nose 6 Parallel-arm step-up 3 × 20	GH training: 5 cycles of :30/:30 1. Alternating high pull 2. High pull to press 3. Squat to press Legs: Step-up 5 × 20 with weight

growth hormone (GH) levels (Gladden 2004; Godfrey, Madgwick, and Whyte 2003; Kraemer and Ratamess 2003). This type of work is essential for female athletes because it changes body composition and enhances power endurance. The exercises for the growth hormone work emphasize movements of the large muscle groups in the whole body. During this block there were no major competitions. This block also included Thanksgiving break and final exams. Because of this, the work is very focused and intense; it is not long and drawn out. Note that the effectiveness of this phase is dependent on the accumulation of training from the previous two phases of training.

In the actual GH workout, the goal is to get as many reps as possible. There are specified goals in terms of reps for each exercise. Once those are achieved, weight must be added. The intensity must never be compromised. The net effect of the GH workout is a significant lactate buildup and immediate general fatigue. There seems to be no residual negative effect on the subsequent swimming workouts. In fact, some of the athletes felt a positive effect. (I think this is caused by a positive endocrine response in female swimmers, but as yet I have no research to prove this.)

The upper-body work was continued with no attempt to raise the volume during this phase. The overall volume was close to the same as for the previous phase, but the intensity and perceived exertion in this phase were significantly higher. This only shows the strength training portion of the dryland program. Core strength modules were also included every day.

Figure 10.4
FOUNDATIONAL STRENGTH

Exercise	Sets	Reps	Comments
Monday			
Dumbbell snatch	4	6	
Dumbbell high pull	2	6	
Dumbbell split jerk	4	6	
Squat to press	3	6	
Squat	5	20	Sandbag or weight vest for resistance
Regular step-up	2	10	Sandbag or weight vest for resistance
Medicine-ball power throws	1		
Single-leg squat and throw		20	10 reps each leg
Single-leg squat and scoop throw		20	10 reps each leg
Squat and throw		10	
Over-the-back throw		10	
Forward through the legs		10	
Thursday			
Dumbbell high pull	4	6	
Dumbbell snatch	2	6	
Dumbbell split jerk	2	6	
Lunge and press	3	6	Anterior lunge
Lunge and reach	5	18	3 reps forward, side, rotational
Step-up (lateral)	2	20	Sandbag or weight vest for resistance
Medicine-ball power throws	1		
Single-leg squat and throw		20	10 reps each leg
Single-leg squat and scoop throw		20	10 reps each leg
Squat and throw		10	
Over-the-back throw		10	
Forward through the legs		10	

Tuesday and Friday			
Incline push-up	5	12	2 regular grip, 2 reverse, 1 rotation
Combo I: curl and press	3	16	8 reps each arm
Incline pull-up	5	12	
Dumbbell row	3	8	8 reps each arm
Front pulldown	3	8	
Arm step-up	2	20	Use 4-inch (10 cm) box or a step
Punching (stretch cord)	2	20	
Overhead throw	1	20	
Soccer throw	1	20	
Chest pass	1	20	
Standing side to side	1	20	10 each side (cross in front)
Standing cross in front	1	20	10 each side
Around the back	1	20	10 each side

Figure 10.5

BASIC STRENGTH

Exercise	Sets	Reps	Comments
Monday			
Dumbbell complex	5		1 minute of recovery between each
Dumbbell high pull		6	
Dumbbell alternating press		6	
Dumbbell squat		6	
Dumbbell row		6	
Leg circuit	5		Progress to no rest between circuits
Squat		20	
Lunge		20	10 reps each leg
Step-up		20	10 reps each leg
Squat jump		10	

(continued)

Figure 10.5 *(continued)*

Exercise	Sets	Reps	Comments
Monday *(continued)*			
Medicine-ball power throws	1		
Single-leg squat and throw		20	10 reps each leg
Single-leg squat and scoop throw		20	10 reps each leg
Squat and throw		10	
Over-the-back throw		10	
Forward through the legs		10	
Tuesday and Friday			
Incline push-up	4	20	2 reps regular grip, 2 reps reverse, 1 rep rotation
Incline pull-up	4	20	
Dumbbell row	5	4	Each arm
Front pulldown	3	4	Go heavy!
Arm step-up	2	20	Use 4-inch (10 cm) box or a step
Punching (stretch cord)	2	20	
Medicine-ball wall throws	2		
Overhead throw		20	
Soccer throw		20	
Chest pass		20	
Standing side to side		20	10 each side (cross in front)
Standing cross in front		20	10 each side
Around the back		20	10 each side
Thursday			
Dumbbell complex II	5		1 minute of recovery between each
Dumbbell snatch		12	6 each arm
Push jerk		6	
Jump shrug		6	
Overhead squat	3	6	
Medicine-ball total-body throws	1		
Contrast	1	10	5 reps with 12-pound (5.5 kg) power ball and 5 reps with 3-kilogram medicine ball
Over the back	1	6	
Forward through the legs	1	6	
Squat throw	1	10	

Strength Endurance

Emphasis: Work in the time range from 30 seconds to 60 seconds with a recovery ratio up to 1:1, but more frequently 1:.33 to 1:.5. See figure 10.6 for specific workouts.

Length of cycle: Three weeks.

Frequency: Three days a week.

Means: Circuit work.

Recycle

Emphasis: Each of the previous components are recycled for short periods to stabilize or refresh those aspects as needed. Figure 10.7 (on page 207) provides specific workouts.

Length of cycle: Three weeks.

Frequency: Three days a week.

Means: Each session will revisit the workout means from the previous cycle.

Hybrid

Emphasis: Each component is covered in a microcycle in order to stabilize strength components in peaking or tapering. See figure 10.8 (on page 208) for specific workouts.

Length of cycle: Three to four weeks.

Frequency: Two or three times a week.

Means: Combination of each of the previous methods.

Figure 10.6

STRENGTH ENDURANCE

Exercise	Sets	Reps	Comments
Monday: general circuit			
Push-up	1	15	
Standing rotation	1	20	
Rotational push-up	1	12	6 each side
2-position sit-up	1	20	10 each side
Standing bench press	1	20	
Medicine-ball chops	1	20	10 each side
Medicine-ball chest pass	1	20	
Stretch-cord Nordic Row	1	20	
Stretch-cord punching	1	20	

(continued)

Figure 10.6 *(continued)*

Exercise	Sets	Reps	Comments
Wednesday: jump rope circuit			
Sandbag high pull	1	12	
Stretch cord: big circle	1	20	10 each direction
High step-up	1	20	10 each leg
Jump rope	1		30 seconds
Incline push-up	1	15	
Stability-ball sit-up	1	20	
Squat	1	20	
Jump rope	1		30 seconds
Alternating press	1	20	10 each arm
Stability-ball pushback	1	20	
Lunge	1	20	
Jump rope	1		30 seconds
Standing bench press	1	20	
Landmine rotations	1	20	10 each side
Step-up	1	30	
Jump rope	1		30 seconds
Curl and press	1	10	
Swim trainer	1	20	
Lateral step-up	1	20	
Jump rope			30 seconds
Arm step-ups	1	20	
Over the top	1	20	
Lateral bound	1	20	10 each side
Jump rope	1		30 seconds
Friday: super seven circuit			
Squat jump	1	10	
Chinnie	1	20	
Push-up	1	20	
Step-up	1	20	
Medicine-ball sit-up	1	20	
Medicine-ball squat and throw	1	20	
Walking lunge	1	20	10 each leg

Figure 10.7
RECYCLE

Exercise	Sets	Reps	Comments
Monday			
Dumbbell high pull	4	4	
Dumbbell snatch	2	4	
Dumbbell split jerk	2	4	
Spectrum squat	3	20	6 reps with sandbag or weight vest followed immediately by 6 fast body-weight squats followed immediately by 8 squat jumps
Lunge and press	3	18	3 reps each position: forward, side, rotational
Incline pull-up	5	15	
Dumbbell row	4	4	Each arm
Front pulldown	3	4	Go heavy!
Arm step-up	2	20	Use 4-inch (10 cm) box or a step
Medicine-ball power throws	1		
Single-leg squat and throw		20	10 reps each leg
Single-leg squat and scoop throw		20	10 reps each leg
Squat and throw		10	
Over-the-back throw		10	
Forward through the legs		10	
Wednesday			
Incline push-up	5	15	2 regular grip, 2 reverse, 1 rotation
Combo I: curl and press	3	16	8 reps each arm
Incline pull-up	3	15	Use weight vest for resistance
Dumbbell row	4	8	4 reps each arm
Front pulldown	3	4	Go heavy!
Arm step-up	2	20	Use 4-inch (10 cm) box or a step
Punching (stretch cord)	2	20	
Friday			
Dumbbell complex	5		1 minute of recovery between each
Alternating dumbbell high pull		6	
Curl and press		12	6 reps each arm
Dumbbell squat		6	
Dumbbell one-arm row		6	
Leg circuit	5		1 minute of recovery between each
Squat		20	
Lunge		20	10 reps each leg
Step-up		20	10 reps each leg
Squat jump		10	

Figure 10.8
HYBRID

Exercise	Sets	Reps	Comments
Monday: maximum power training			
Dumbbell high pull	3	4	Alternative: high pull throw with sandbag
Dumbbell one-arm snatch	3	4	Alternative: snatch throw with powerball
Push jerk	2	6	Alternative: jerk throw with 8-kg medicine ball
Squat jump	3	10	Descending loading: heavy sandbag, medium sandbag, no sandbag
Hurdle stiffness jumps	5	4	
Thursday			
Dumbbell high pull	2	4	
Dumbbell one-arm snatch	4	2	
Push jerk	2	4	
Squat jump	3	10	Use big band
Hurdle stiffness jumps	5	10	

SUMMARY

In a sound strength training program, the work must incorporate multiple joints in the exercises. Strength is literally built from the ground up with the emphasis on the lower extremities to prepare athletes to optimize ground reaction forces. Strength and stability of the core are the cornerstone of the program. All training is core training. The program must incorporate balance and proprioception and include pulling movements, pressing (pushing) movements, squat movements, and derivatives to integrate the whole kinetic chain and reinforce linkage.

The goals of the strength training program should align to the sport the athletes are preparing for. One program is not suitable for all sports and all athletes. Understand how programs differ based on the objectives. It is possible for the exercises to be the same, but manipulation of sets, reps, rest, and load can significantly change the training effect.

Integrated Power Training

Plyometric training is not a stand-alone training method. It is an important part of a bigger picture, the logical culmination of the strength training spectrum because of its high speed and high force. It is certainly a supporting structure to speed training and a key aspect of rehabilitation. As a training method plyometrics has been misunderstood. Much of the misunderstanding arises from the belief that it is a stand-alone method. In order for plyometric training to be most effective, it must be integrated into a complete training program.

Plyometrics is not a secret Eastern European training method as it has sometimes been portrayed. It simply takes advantage of the naturally occurring stretch–shortening cycle of muscle action, which is an integral part of movement. Jumping, hopping, and bounding activities are natural activities. They are part of the normal play of children. The systematic approach to the use of plyometric training was probably pioneered in track and field in the jumping events in preparation for performance. I prefer to narrow the scope of the training method to jumping, hopping, and bounding movements and activities that involve projection of the center of mass either horizontally or vertically in order to increase the magnitude and rate of stretch on the muscles. I prefer not to use the term *upper-body plyometrics*, which is encompassed in core training and strength training for the upper body.

PLYOMETRIC TRAINING FUNDAMENTALS

Plyometric training is based on training the stretch–shortening cycle of muscle action to enhance the subsequent concentric action. The use of the stretch–shortening cycle is essential for efficient human movement. It is a quality of muscle action that is highly trainable and adaptable. Over the years much confusion and mythology have arisen about this method of training. The word *plyometrics* first appeared in coaching literature in the late 1960s, and the misconception arose that it was then that the system was first used. That is definitely not the case. Jumping, hopping, and bounding activities have been used throughout the ages, although it was not until the mid-20th century that these activities were systematically applied to athletic performance enhancement. It is scientifically accurate and more descriptive to call this method elastic, or reactive training, but that is a cumbersome term; hence the term *plyometrics* is more commonly used. Reactive training is certainly more descriptive of the goals of the training method and the physiological demands, because essentially the athlete is training the elastic properties of the muscle to be more reactive to the ground.

The goals of plyometric training are threefold: to raise explosive power, to learn to better attenuate ground reaction forces regardless of the event or sport, and to learn to be able to tolerate and use greater stretch loads (in essence to increase muscle stiffness). The last point demands a bit more explanation. Musculotendinous stiffness is the key to reactive training. It is highly related to the body's ability to store and reuse elastic energy from running and jumping. The concept of stiffness is sometimes confusing because we tend to equate stiffness with a lack of flexibility, but for explosive movements this is not the case. A stiff muscle will develop a high degree of tension as it is stretched. This is very desirable for raising explosiveness. Conversely, a muscle that lacks stiffness will collapse and absorb elastic energy. It does not react as actively to the ground; therefore, it will produce significantly less explosiveness. Think of sagging as the opposite of stiffness. A simple analogy to help you understand stiffness is the comparison of a soft rubber playground ball to a golf ball. If both balls were dropped onto a hard concrete surface, the golf ball would react rapidly and bounce high; the playground ball, on the other hand, would react slowly to the ground and not bounce as high. In plyometric training, to optimize ground reaction forces, you want to stimulate the golf ball–type reaction. A stiff muscle is able to produce optimal amounts of reactive force in a short period. This is why the rate of stretch is so important in eliciting a positive training response.

Plyometric training is highly compatible with and significantly enhanced by strength training. It is also closely related to speed development. Most important, it is *not* a conditioning tool! Because of the explosive nature of the work, it is of high neural demand; therefore, it should not be used for conditioning. It should almost never be trained in a climate of fatigue, with a few notable exceptions. Those exceptions are sports that demand power endurance, such as soccer, rugby, basketball, 400-meter race or 400-meter hurdles, and 800 meters. Even in those sports the fatigue element is introduced only after the technical component of the exercise is mastered. This will minimize risk of injury. The stimulus for adaptation is not volume; it is intensity. Never compromise the intensity of the movements. Too much emphasis has been placed on volume in terms of the number of contacts. This was certainly a mistake I made in my early years of coaching. A typical session then was 300 to 400 contacts! Did I get good results? Yes, but I think it was in spite of the training, not because of the training. The athletes were gifted and had a good training background, so they were able to tolerate the work.

Remember that training is not just tolerating the work. It is eliciting a positive adaptive response. As I have learned more of the science of plyometrics and how it fits with the other components of training, I have modified the approach. I have significantly reduced the number of contacts in a training session and a microcycle. Today a high-volume session is in the range of 90 to 120 contacts with a range of 250 to 400 contacts for a seven-day microcycle. More is definitely not better. If used properly, it is an effective tool in stimulating the nervous system. But if used improperly, it can have the opposite effect and dull, if not deaden, the nervous system. Consider the load with respect to the other components of training.

Plyometric training consists of three basic movements. The most fundamental plyometric activity is jumping, which is characterized by two-foot landings. The jump is the least stressful activity because on landing body weight is distributed over both legs. Hopping is characterized by one-foot landings. Hops are the most stressful because all landing forces are absorbed on one leg. Bounding is characterized by alternate-leg landing and subsequent takeoffs. The bound is more stressful than jumping but not as stressful as hopping because landing forces are alternated off one leg onto the other leg. This provides very specific guidance on how to progress and distribute work as well as how to integrate plyometric training with the other components of training. The complexity in plyometric training comes from combining these movements and their derivatives.

To thoroughly understand plyometric training, you need to understand jumping mechanics. First, to maximize power production, it is necessary to use as many joints as possible to produce force. This results in a summation of forces, which produces the highest ground reaction forces possible. A good way to represent this is what Kreighbaum and Barthels (1995) have called the spring model (see figure 11.1). Imagine that there is a set of springs at the ankle, the knee, and the hip. To achieve maximum force production, you need to compress all those springs and then sequentially release that tension, resulting in triple extension of the ankle, knee, and hip to produce the height of the jump. Another contributing factor is the transfer of momentum from one body segment to another. As one segment begins to slow down, the momentum from that segment is transferred to the next segment and on up the chain. The ultimate result is the body applying force against the ground; this is called ground reaction force. Application of force against the ground in order to jump high or far is the result of all segments of the body contributing to the force production. The largest segmental contribution comes from the lower extremities, then the trunk, then the arms, and, even at the end, extension of the neck and head. All of this demands a high degree of coordination to sum up the forces and then apply that force to achieve optimal results.

Landing mechanics are the opposite of takeoff mechanics. Use as many joints as possible to reduce force on landing. Sequentially bend the ankle, the knee, and the hip. If no subsequent takeoff is required, then the flexion should be relatively deep to absorb shock. If a rapid subsequent takeoff is required, then the joints should bend only as much as necessary to load the muscles to produce force for the subsequent jump. Remember the concept of stiffness.

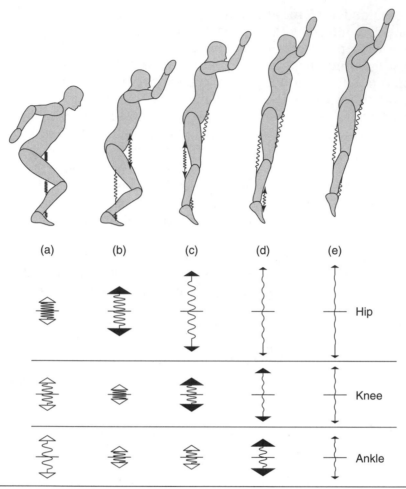

Figure 11.1   Spring model of the body segments in a jump. The spring model illustrates the elasticity of the muscles by drawing an analogy to springs crossing the ankle, knee, and hip. Compressing these springs will result in the subsequent elastic rebound.

Fig. 12.19, p. 408 from BIOMECHANICS by Ellen Kreighbaum and Katharine M. Bartels. Copyright © 1981 by Burgess Publishing Company. Reprinted by permission of Pearson Education, Inc.

PLYOMETRICS PHASES

Some additional terminology will further clarify and facilitate communication and understanding. The plyometric action is broken down into phases. All plyometric activity is initiated with an amortization phase, also called the *yielding phase.* This is the lowering, or eccentric, phase of the movement. This puts the muscle on a stretch and loads the muscle. When the end of the phase is reached, the key to plyometric training occurs. This is the switching time, or coupling time, where the rapid switch from eccentric to concentric work occurs. Essentially it is this switching time that you are training. The faster that you can get athletes to switch from eccentric to concentric action, the more explosive the athletes will be. Ultimately plyometric training is focused on enhancing the capabilities of rapid switching from eccentric to concentric muscle action in ballistic movements.

The prerequisites for effective application of plyometric training are coordination, balance, body control, and awareness. Core control and core strength are also very important in maintaining good dynamic posture during the movements. Leg strength relative to the level of the athlete's development is a must. It is not necessary to be able to squat a certain amount of weight; rather it is necessary to exhibit a high degree of functional leg strength. If these prerequisites are at an acceptable level, then the athlete is ready to start a basic progression. Progression is essential in minimizing injury and optimizing training adaptation. Lead-up activities done in a gamelike environment are an important part of progression as well as good preparation. Games such as hopscotch, sack races, and jumps for distance are tremendous preparation for the formal training to follow.

The balance progression (see chapter 8) and mastery of these steps will go a long way toward making plyometric training a lower-risk, high-return training method. Dynamic and ballistic balance work tunes up the nervous system as well as emphasizes good landing mechanics and posture, which are the keys to successful use of plyometric training. The key to progression is to teach landing first. Jim Radcliffe, strength and conditioning coach at the University of Oregon, stresses that how you land determines how you take off. Regardless of the level of athlete, this must be emphasized and reinforced in each plyometric session. Proper foot position is essential in effective landings. The landing is on a full foot (mid-foot contact), not on the ball of the foot or a completely flat foot. A mid-foot landing will set the foot up in a position to absorb shock and make better use of the elasticity of the muscles up the kinetic chain. This will set up an athlete's readiness for any subsequent takeoffs on multiple-response activities. After athletes have mastered landing, teach the takeoff, which is a triple extension of ankle, knee, and hip—the summation of forces. As mentioned previously, the balance progression certainly reinforces good landing mechanics, and since balance work can be incorporated easily into an active warm-up, it enables you to accomplish a two-pronged training effect: improving balance and reinforcing landing mechanics daily. I have found that working barefoot on forgiving surfaces such as gymnastics floor exercise mats teaches athletes how to use their feet properly in landing.

The common denominator in all plyometric exercises is projection of the center of gravity. Therefore, plyometric training is classified descriptively based on the projection of the center of gravity. The in-place response is characterized by vertical displacement of the center of gravity coupled with short contact times. The short response is characterized by horizontal displacement of the center of gravity with 10 contacts or fewer. The long response is characterized by horizontal displacement of the center of gravity with speed and more than 10 contacts. To get a better command of putting the classifications into a coherent program, the plyometric demand matrix (see figure 11.2) was developed to govern progression. The progression variables can be manipulated by moving down the column or across. The suggested range of sets, repetitions, and distance appears in each row.

For the athlete of advanced training age, the numbers can be pushed up slightly as long as quality is not compromised. Keep in mind that this matrix is only a rough guideline and must be adapted to fit the sport and the individual athlete.

Plyometric training can be used two or three times in a seven-day microcycle depending on the phase of the year and the sport. Low-amplitude, remedial in-place movements can be done daily as part of a warm-up. Start with simple movements in place and then add combinations as the athletes achieve mastery. As for sequence and compatibility with other components, plyometric training and strength training are very complementary. Plyometric training is also very compatible with speed development. Given this fundamental compatibility with other methods of high neural demand, it is imperative to take into account the overall stress on the nervous system when combining methods. In the training spectrum, plyometric training is at the high-speed, high-force ballistic end of the spectrum. The number of contacts, the type of exercise, and the complexity change as the season progresses and with the level of development of the athlete. It is best to work on this early in the workout before any fatigue sets in. With younger developing athletes, put plyometric training before strength training and before sprinting. As athletes advance in training age, plyometric work can be combined with strength training during certain phases and even follow strength training. Table 11.1 shows such a combination that I used with a high school girls' basketball team in their fifth month of training. This workout occurred in the late preseason period. The sequence is very dependent on training age.

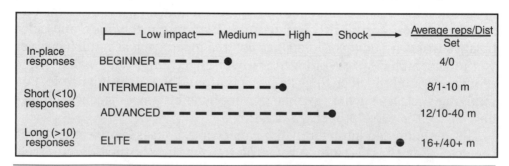

Figure 11.2 Plyometric demand matrix.

Reprinted, by permission, from J. Radcliffe and R. Farentinos, 1999, *High-powered plyometrics* (Champaign, IL: Human Kinetics), 42. Adapted from V.R. Gambetta, R. Rogers, R. Fields, D. Semenick and J. Radcliffe, 1986, NSCA Plyometric Videotape Symposium, Lincoln, NE.

Table 11.1 Elastic Equivalent Workout*

	Strength exercise	Plyometric exercise
Pair 1	Dumbbell snatch × 10 each arm	Hurdle jumps 2 × 5 (21 to 30 inches, or 51 to 76 centimeters)
Pair 2	Dumbbell high pull × 10 each arm	Jump-up × 1
Pair 3	Squat × 10	Squat jump × 10 (with arms)
Pair 4	Side lunge with dumbbells × 10	BOSU lateral bound 2 × 10 each side
Pair 5	Lateral step-up (sandbag) × 10	Lateral jump × 12 (over 12-inch [30-centimeter] obstacle)

*Each pair couples a strength exercise with a plyometric exercise. Complete 2 sets of each pair. Allow three minutes rest between pairs of exercise to ensure explosiveness.

When problems do occur with plyometric training, it is often because of a lack of progression, too much too soon, or an inappropriate selection of exercises. Also poor technique in the actual execution of the exercises can create inappropriate stress. Strength deficiencies either in the lower extremities or the core coupled with the previous two deficiencies can be a major factor in injury. Use plyometric training progressively, and always consider it in context with the whole training program.

Plyometrics Teaching Progression

Following a methodical teaching progression will minimize the risk of injury and maximize the return. The plyometric teaching progression is a multistep process. The progression is based on criteria. Mastery of each step is necessary for progression to the next step. The first three steps may be accomplished within the first teaching or training session. All of step 4 should be mastered in the second session, or it should be repeated until the movements are mastered. The beauty of this progression is that you will be able to quickly identify faults and deficiencies before they become a problem. Then you can address and correct the deficiencies early in the stages of learning before they become ingrained. The progression is also an evaluative tool.

❶ Landing

Goal: Teach proper foot strike; use of ankle, knee, and hip; and correct body alignment.

- Step and catch. Walk forward, stepping onto one foot. Land on a flat foot with a slight flexion of the ankle, knee, and hip; hold. Repeat with other foot. Do this three to five times on each foot until foot strike on landing is mastered.

- Step down off a low box (2 to 6 inches, or 5 to 15 centimeters). Step down onto one foot and land on a flat foot with slight flexion of the ankle, knee, and hip; hold. Repeat with other foot.
- Execute a standing long jump (submaximal) with the emphasis on "sticking" the landing. Land quietly on a full foot, and absorb shock by bending the ankle, knee, and hip. Check on landing that the hips are over the feet and the chest is over the knees. Repeat several times until comfortable.
- Hop out onto one foot. This should be a submaximal effort with the emphasis on sticking the landing. Land quietly on a full foot, and absorb shock by bending the ankle, knee, and hip. Check on landing that the hips are over the feet and the chest is over the knees. Repeat several times until comfortable.

❷ Stabilization responses

Goal: To reinforce correct landing technique, raise levels of eccentric strength, and improve ability to stabilize.

- Execute a standing long jump. Hold the landing position for five counts.
- Hop out onto one foot.

Repeat the exercise until the athlete is able to stick and hold three hops on each leg for five counts. If the athlete is a multidirectional sport athlete it would be appropriate to include lateral and rotational jumps and hops to assess ability in multiple planes. This is not only a performance indicator but also an injury-prevention indicator.

❸ Jump-up

Goal: To teach the takeoff action; triple extension of the ankle, knee, and hip joints; and efficient use of the arms.

- Start with a stable bench or box that is knee height. Jump up onto the box. Emphasize a forceful swing of the arms to transfer momentum to the whole body.
- Progress to mid-thigh height.

Eventually the athlete should be able to progress comfortably to jumps up to waist height.

❹ In-place responses

Goal: To teach quick reaction on and off the ground and vertical displacement of the center of gravity.

- Begin by reviewing the first three steps. This will serve as a good warm-up as well as a review of the concepts.
- Execute a bouncing movement in the ankles. The knees repetitively jump in place by using plantar flexion of the ankles.
- Execute a tuck jump, emphasizing quick reaction off the ground while bringing the knees to the chest. Keep the torso erect.

- Execute a scissor jump as a lead-up to the cycle jump, which consists of a jump with a cycling action of the legs.

During the tuck jump check to see if the athlete has the balance and body control to stay in one place. If the athlete is unable to land and take off in a small area, this is a sign of poor body control. Do not progress until the athlete is able to achieve balance and body control.

❺ Short responses

Goal: To teach horizontal displacement of the center of gravity.

- Review the previous steps.
- Begin with repeat standing long jumps. Start with two consecutive jumps (two-foot takeoff and landing) and progress to five consecutive standing long jumps.
- Do repetitive stair jumps (five repeat jumps on stairs).
- Do a single-leg hop. Work up to 10 consecutive hops on each leg.

On the single-leg hops, emphasize the cyclic action of both the active hopping leg and the free leg. The action should resemble a single-leg run. Repeat step 5 for two workouts before progressing to the next step.

❻ Long responses

Goal: To add horizontal velocity.

- Begin with high skips, emphasizing projection up and out.
- Do alternate leg bounding, carried out for 10 to 20 contacts.
- Do combinations of hops and bounds, carried out for 10 to 20 contacts.

This is as far as most athletes should progress in the first year of training. It is possible to increase the volume, intensity, and complexity of the workouts by adding exercises and combinations of exercises in the six steps.

❼ Shock method

Goal: High nervous system demand. This is an advanced form of training that requires a large training base.

- Execute jumps down from boxes or rebound jumps over hurdles placed at mid-thigh height or higher.

The training stress is high; therefore, this method should be used judiciously. The shock method is inappropriate for beginners.

Several key teaching concepts will serve to reinforce correct mechanics and the objectives of the training progression:

- Landing (key word is *bending*). Remember that how you land determines how you take off. Use as many joints as possible to reduce force.
- Take-off (key word is *extending*). Use triple extension of the ankle, knee, and hip. Use as many joints as possible to produce force.

- Use the ground (key words are *the ground is hot*). Use two-foot landings, one-foot landings, and alternate-foot landings.
- Get vertical (key word is *up*). Project and displace up.
- Get horizontal (key word is *out*). Project and displace out.

PLYOMETRICS PROGRAM DESIGN CONSIDERATIONS

In order for plyometric training to be effective, you must consider specific aspects in program design. Athletes need to display technical proficiency in performing the exercises. Poor technique will lead to inefficient application of force and, if repeated enough, it will cause injury. Consider the weight of each athlete in the selection of exercises and in assignment of volume of jumps. Heavier athletes will be under more stress simply from the effects of gravity. I have always used this guideline: If a male athlete is over 190 pounds (86 kilograms) and if a female athlete is over 150 pounds (68 kilograms), then make adjustments in the exercise selection and volume of contacts. In designing the workout, consider the displacement of the center of gravity. I usually have a vertical emphasis on one day and a horizontal emphasis on another day. Responses to vertical displacement seem to be more stressful, and responses to horizontal displacement are less stressful. Remember too that single-support (one-leg) activities are significantly more stressful than double-support (two-leg) activities, so be sure to take this into account when designing a workout. I like to start with some basic double-support jumps to tune up the nervous system before moving to single-support actions. Consider the speed as well; higher-speed movements are more stressful.

I have not found it beneficial or even necessary to add external load to plyometric activities. External load slows the action, which is counterproductive to the high-speed, high-force objective of plyometric training. The only exception to this is loaded squat jumps, which by their very nature are a slower movement. Training age has a significant impact on program design. At younger training ages the complexity of the exercises should be kept considerably lower. As the athletes progress, complexity can increase, as can the volume of loading. Choose stable shoes for plyometric training. Do not be fooled into thinking that the shoes can make up for poor landing mechanics. The midsole of the shoes should not be too spongy, because this causes instability and actually creates more problems than it solves. Barefoot training can be good on a floor exercise mat or even in sand. A proper training surface will minimize the risk in plyometric training. Choose a firm, forgiving surface. Smooth grass is best. Concrete or asphalt should not be used. A sprung gym floor or an aerobics floor works quite well. Too soft a surface will take away from the elastic response and make the action more concentric in nature, so consider that in the selection of the surface.

Remember that volume is not the stimulus for adaptation in plyometric training. Keep the volume relatively low and the intensity high. Adding fatigue will compromise quality. Seldom if ever would I recommend exceeding 150 contacts in a training session, unless they are low-amplitude remedial bouncing movements such as those that occur in jumping rope. Seldom is plyometric training done on two consecutive training days. Because of the neural demand, it is necessary to allow time for recovery. Generally 48 hours is required. Low-level, remedial plyometric activities can be done daily as an injury-prevention routine as long as they are carefully sequenced with the overall workload. Typically plyometric work is prescribed in sets and reps of a particular exercise. That is fine, but do not get so enamored with it that you neglect to evaluate the quality of each exercise. Make sure that the technique is good. Do not hesitate to end the exercise or even the whole plyometric session if you see the quality decline. A good indicator is the sound of the contacts. Loud, percussive contacts usually are an indicator that it is time to end the exercise. Intraworkout recovery is also important. Take adequate time between sets to ensure quality of movement. In a team setting, put the players in lines and let that dictate recovery time. Longer lines allow more recovery.

Integration With Strength Training

The integration of plyometrics and strength training is a natural fit. They are mutually beneficial. The following are some general considerations that are somewhat dependent on training age: when to lift, when to jump, when to lift and jump, and when to jump and lift. At the younger training ages it is best to lift after plyometric training. The opposite is true at more advanced training ages. At advanced training ages a low-volume, explosive lifting session followed by a low-volume, high-intensity plyometric session can significantly enhance the plyometric workout. Generally at the early training ages, it is not best to mix lifting and plyometrics. Achieving optimal benefit from this combination requires a good work capacity base that takes several years to acquire. At advanced training the judicious combination of lifting and plyometrics can be very beneficial in exciting the nervous system and raising explosive power. A cautionary note here is warranted: Even at advanced training ages, do not overdo the combination of lifting and plyometrics. When used in short, sharp, concentrated blocks, lifting and plyometrics can raise explosive power; when carried out for too long, this combination has the opposite effect.

Playlike Plyometrics for Young Athletes

There is some controversy regarding plyometric training for young athletes. There is no physiological reason why young developing athletes cannot do plyometric training. First, remember that plyometric training, by its very nature, is a very natural activity. Children at play are always jumping, hopping, and bounding—remember hopscotch? Therefore, for young athletes, the more playlike and natural the plyometric activities, the better the training effect. Hopping races and jumping games will accomplish the desired training effect. Make it as instinctual as possible. Incorporate a task that will elicit the desired plyometric response. Give young athletes targets to hit with repetitive hops. Put a circle on the ground and require them to land in each circle with a different foot on each contact and gradually increase the distance of the circles, which will teach bounding. Higher-level, more formal training can come with advanced training ages.

Specific Sport Context

There are certainly sport-specific considerations in regard to plyometric training. I have found that in sports in which athletes are on their feet for extended periods, plyometric training must be used judiciously. In these types of sports, the majority of the plyometric work should be concentrated in the off-season. In a sport such as volleyball, where jumping is inherent in the game, adding the additional stress of extensive plyometric training can have a negative effect, especially during the in-season. It can add needless fatigue, which predisposes athletes to injury. The bottom line is to assess the impact forces that already exist in the sport you are coaching. If it is high, then you must carefully select the methods, volume, and intensity of plyometric training. Plyometric training is appropriate for virtually any sport if properly applied in the context of the sport. Remember that the goals of plyometric training are to raise explosive power, better attenuate ground reaction forces, and learn to tolerate stretch loads. There is not a sport that could not profit from one or all three of the goals.

SAMPLE PLYOMETRIC TRAINING PROGRAM

Table 11.2 on pages 224 through 226 provides a six-week progressive program designed for high school athletes. The assumption in this program is that the athletes will do nothing but jump and strength train during this time. The strength training program is not detailed here, but you should apply the principles spelled out in the previous chapter. The athletes should do no endurance work during this program aside from playing the sport.

The first four exercises are remedial in nature; therefore, they are done during each session as a specific warm-up for the more complex exercises to follow. Each of these exercises reinforces the basics of plyometrics while warming up the athletes for the more intense work to follow. Watch these exercises and make sure they are executed with precision. Just because they are done daily and classified as remedial does not make them any less important.

- **Jump rope.** Basic double-leg jumps in sets of 25 repetitions.
- **Multidirectional jumps.** Jump forward, side, opposite side, back, and repeat. Keep contact time short.

- **Jump and stick.** Jump out and land, flexing the ankles, knees, and hips. Stick the landing and hold for five counts.

- **Hop and stick.** Same as the previous exercise but take off and land on one leg.

- **Hurdle jump.** Take off from two feet and land. Then jump up over the next hurdle (figure 11.3). This involves vertical projection of the center of gravity, so it can be stressful. Start with 1 hurdle and progress up to 10 hurdles. For beginners, start with the hurdles at 18 inches (46 centimeters) and progress in 3-inch (8-centimeter) increments until they are up 30 inches (76 centimeters). If the hurdle is too high, then ground contact time will increase, which defeats the purpose of the drill.

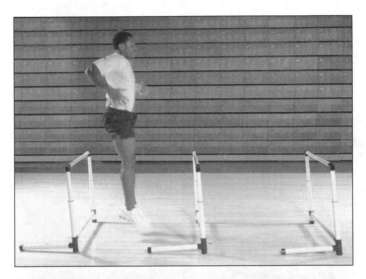

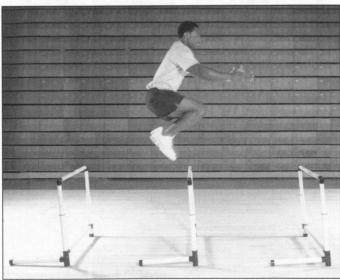

Figure 11.3 Hurdle jump.

- **Squat jump.** Quickly squat down and jump up as high as possible. Do not use the arms. Keep the hands on the hips in order to force triple extension of the ankles, knees, and hips. This is also used in testing, so it is specific preparation for testing. It is appropriate to add loading to this exercise as long as speed is not compromised. The best method of loading that does not interfere with the movement would be a weight vest or a sandbag. Start with 10 percent of body weight and gradually progress to 20 percent body weight as the athlete adapts.

- **Double-leg jump.** Jump out as far as possible and repeat continuously for the prescribed number of jumps. This involves horizontal displacement. Project out and up and emphasize being quick off the ground. These are sometimes called frog jumps, which is descriptive of the motion.

- **Band jump.** With a rubber band draped over the shoulders, the movement is the same as the squat jump. The rubber band should be firmly anchored to the ground or a piece of heavy equipment, or a partner can stand on the band to provide consistent resistance (figure 11.4). This will accentuate the eccentric component of the jumping action.

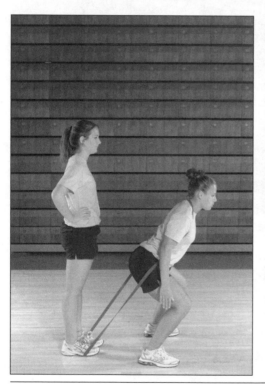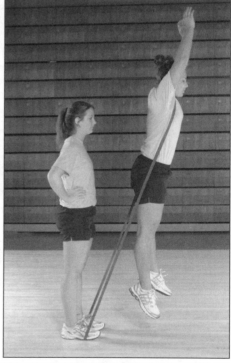

Figure 11.4 Band jump.

- **Vertical jump.** Jump for maximum height using the arms to reach as high as possible. This is a basic testing movement that is also used in training.

- **Step–close jump.** Start with one foot forward; with the other foot, step forward onto two feet and jump up as high as possible using the arms. This demands high coordination because it involves converting horizontal energy into vertical energy. This is a common jumping movement in basketball and volleyball.

- **Jump-up.** Jump up onto a box or a bench. Emphasize great extension of the ankles, knees, and hips and a big arm swing (figure 11.5). Start with a box at knee height, progress to mid-thigh height, to waist height, and possibly to chest height. This exercise reinforces triple extension of the ankles, knees, and hips, a key movement for success in sports. It is especially good for bigger, heavier athletes because the emphasis is on the jump up onto to something. This minimizes landing forces by cheating gravity.

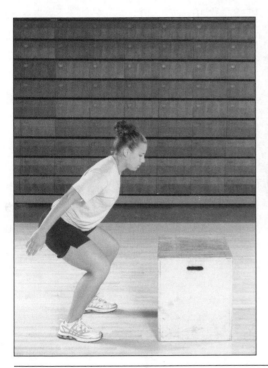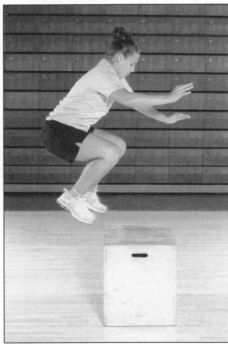

Figure 11.5 Jump-up.

Table 11.2 Six-Week Plyometrics Training Program

Week 1									
	Day 1			Day 2			Day 3		
Exercise	Sets	Reps	Volume	Sets	Reps	Volume	Sets	Reps	Volume
Jump rope	3	25	75	4	25	100	5	25	125
Jump and stick	1	10	10	1	10	10	1	10	10
Hop and stick	1	10	10	1	10	10	1	10	10
Multidirectional jumps	2	8	16	2	8	16	2	8	16
Jump-up (knee height)	2	10	20	3	10	30	4	10	40
Hurdle jump 24 inches (60 cm)	5	5	25						
Double-leg jump for distance				3	5	15			
Band jump				3	10	30	4	8	32
Squat jump	3	12	36				3	15	45
Jump volume per session			192			211			278
Jump volume per week									681

Week 2									
	Day 1			Day 2			Day 3		
Exercise	Sets	Reps	Volume	Sets	Reps	Volume	Sets	Reps	Volume
Jump rope	3	25	75	4	25	100	5	25	125
Jump and stick	1	10	10	1	10	10	1	10	10
Hop and stick	1	10	10	1	10	10	1	10	10
Multidirectional jumps	2	8	16	2	8	16	2	8	16
Jump-up (knee height)	3	5	15				2	5	10
Vertical jump				3	5	15			
Hurdle jump 24 inches (60 cm)	5	10	50						
Double-leg jump				5	5	25			
Band jump				4	10	40	5	8	40
Squat jump	3	18	54				3	21	63
Jump volume per session			230			216			274
Jump volume per week									720

Week 3									
	Day 1			Day 2			Day 3		
Exercise	Sets	Reps	Volume	Sets	Reps	Volume	Sets	Reps	Volume
Jump rope	3	25	75	4	25	100	5	25	125
Jump and stick	1	10	10	1	10	10	1	10	10
Hop and stick	1	10	10	1	10	10	1	10	10
Multidirectional jumps	2	8	16	2	8	16	2	8	16
Jump-up (thigh height)	3	5	15	3	5	15			
Band jump				5	10	50	5	8	40
Step–close	3	5	15	3	5	15			
Squat jump	3	24	72				3	24	72
Hurdle jump 24 inches (60 cm)	5	10	50						
Double-leg jump				5	5	25			
Jump volume per session			263			241			273
Jump volume per week									777

Week 4									
	Day 1			Day 2			Day 3		
Exercise	Sets	Reps	Volume	Sets	Reps	Volume	Sets	Reps	Volume
Jump rope	3	25	75	4	25	100	5	25	125
Jump and stick	1	10	10	1	10	10	1	10	10
Hop and stick	1	10	10	1	10	10	1	10	10
Multidirectional jumps	2	8	16	2	8	16	2	8	16
Jump-up (thigh height)	3	5	15				3	5	15
Step–close	3	5	15	3	5	15	2	5	10
Vertical jump				3	5	15			
Hurdle jump 24 inches (60 cm)	5	10	50						
Band jump				3	10	30	5	8	40
Double-leg jump				5	5	25			
Squat jump	3	15	45				3	18	54
Jump volume per session			236			221			280
Jump volume per week									737

(continued)

Table 11.2 *(continued)*

Week 5									
	Day 1			Day 2			Day 3		
Exercise	Sets	Reps	Volume	Sets	Reps	Volume	Sets	Reps	Volume
Jump rope	3	25	75	4	25	100	5	25	125
Jump and stick	1	10	10	1	10	10	1	10	10
Hop and stick	1	10	10	1	10	10	1	10	10
Multidirectional jumps	1	8	8	1	8	8	1	8	8
Jump-up (waist height)	3	5	15				3	5	15
Vertical jump				2	5	10			
Step–close	2	5	10	2	5	10			
Hurdle jump 28 inches (70 cm)	5	10	50				5	10	50
Band jump				4	5	20			
Squat jump	3	21	63				3	24	72
Jump volume per session			241			168			290
Jump volume per week									699

Week 6									
	Day 1			Day 2			Day 3		
Exercise	Sets	Reps	Volume	Sets	Reps	Volume	Sets	Reps	Volume
Jump rope	3	25	75	4	25	100	5	25	125
Jump and stick	1	10	10	1	10	10	1	10	10
Hop and stick	1	10	10	1	10	10	1	10	10
Multidirectional jumps	1	8	8	1	8	8	1	8	8
Vertical jump	5	3	15	3	5	15	3	5	15
Step–close	3	3	9						
Jump-up (waist height)				3	5	15			
Hurdle jump 28 inches (70 cm)	2	10	20				2	10	20
Band jump				2	10	20			
Squat jump	3	27	81				3	30	90
Jump volume per session			228			178			278
Jump volume per week									684

SUMMARY

Plyometric training represents the high-speed, high-force end of the strength spectrum. This is the logical culmination of the foundation that athletes acquired through strength training. To ensure the viability of the method, be methodical in the progressions and technically exact in the execution of the exercises.

Linear and Multidimensional Speed

We have all heard the adage "Sprinters are born, not made." This traditional thinking—that an athlete is naturally fast or has no real hope of becoming so—prevails in many circles today. It is true to the extent that it is not possible to be a world-class sprinter without a certain genetic endowment. But few athletes ever reach their true potential in speed. Perhaps that's because as a fine-motor skill, speed takes considerable time to develop to its highest levels. That is especially true of absolute speed, a component the East Germans appropriately called "fast coordination." It is more difficult to develop because it is so dependent on other biomotor qualities—strength, power, flexibility, anaerobic power and capacity, and even aerobic power. While it is tempting to separate speed from those other conditioning components, it is possible for an athlete to achieve maximum speed only in conjunction with the other areas of training. For this reason, this chapter is sequenced as a logical extension to the training of other components in this book.

As a motor skill, with a specific objective in mind, speed can be enhanced by applying principles of motor learning and systematic training. For sprinters the ultimate objective is to achieve maximum velocity and maintain top speed as long as possible through the finish for the fastest possible time. For games players, it involves applying speed to the game.

The demands of speed are significantly different if you are working with a specialist sprinter as opposed to working with an athlete in a multidirectional sport. One fundamental mistake, certainly one that I have made, was to use track-oriented drills and workouts to improve speed for athletes in multidirectional sports. There are different mechanical demands in multidirectional, start-and-stop sports that render most of the traditional track-oriented drills ineffective. The application of speed to sports that require multidirectional movements demands an understanding of the concept of game speed. Game speed is not linear track speed. It is the ability to apply all elements of speed to the demands of the game. Multidirectional sports are not track meets. In fact, some of the technical aspects of speed that are rewarded in the sprint events in track and field can be counterproductive to game speed. Very little movement in multidirectional sports is straight ahead for any significant distance. In straight-ahead speed there is a distinct flight phase that allows the leg to cycle through. In multidirectional movement the flight phase is detrimental to performance. If the feet are not close to the ground it is difficult to change direction and stop. Most movement involves angles, curves, starts, stops, and direction changes. Multidimensional speed and agility and game speed are closely related. MDSA is defined as the ability to recognize, react, start, and move in the required direction, change direction if necessary, and stop quickly. This typically occurs in a time frame of two to five seconds.

To address these differing demands, I developed the 3S system—sport-specific speed. Speed is divided into two major categories: straight-ahead speed (SAS) and multidimensional speed and agility (MDSA). The two are related because all aspects of speed training are derived from the model of the 100-meter sprint. Because world-class competitive sprinters are the fastest human beings, we can conceptually and practically apply what they do to achieve these performances to any activity that demands some component of speed. The principles that apply for the training of the 100-meter sprinters can be adapted to all sports, not just track and field. I emphasize the principles and concepts, not the drills.

STRAIGHT-AHEAD SPEED

To better understand straight-ahead speed and its application, let's look at training for the 100-meter sprint. The 100-meter sprint is the essence of speed, so it is imperative to understand this event in order to understand speed in a broader context. To reinforce the dynamics of sprinting, table 12.1 details the parameters of specific components of the sprint stride. The world record in the 100 meters has improved in large part because of a more systematic and scientific approach to training. A major factor in the improvement was the ability to thoroughly analyze the race by breaking the race into segments.

Zonal Training

I have taken the data of races and adapted them into a concept called zonal training. Division of the sprint into zones provides a context for evaluating the race and logical divisions of the training process. This allows the breakdown of training into manageable parts, and each part has a specific purpose. The zones relate directly to the concept of race distribution. Even though race distribution assumes more importance for elite sprinters because of their strength, race experience, and command of technique, the concept should be introduced at the developmental level as a key element for speed improvement. Each race is broken down into specific zones based on how the athletes run their races. This information is then used in designing the direction of work to improve times in the future. Every race consists of the following four zones:

Table 12.1 Mechanical Dynamics of the 100-Meter Race

Stride length	Initially, short strides increase to moderate and then to longer strides throughout acceleration. In maximum speed, stride length should be maintained.
Ground contact time	This is the amount of time the foot is in contact with the ground. Ground contact time transitions from long ground contacts at the start and early acceleration (as a mechanism to generate force into the ground) to very short ground contacts in the remainder of the race (.22 second→.11 second→.09 second).
Flight time	This is the time spent in the air. Flight time is short during the first few strides of the race, but it becomes longer during the remainder of the race. Short to long (.03 second→.08 second→.119 seconds).
Shin angle to ground	This is the angle between the tibia and the ground. It starts at a very small angle. As stride length increases and body inclination changes, the shin angle to the ground increases to between 70 and 85 degrees.
Trunk angle	In the blocks, trunk angle from the horizontal is large, and the angle increases rapidly at the beginning of the race and then continues to increase gradually until maximum velocity is reached.
Velocity	This is slow at the start of the race and increases rapidly over the first 20 meters. Velocity increases more gradually for the next 30 to 40 meters until maximum velocity is reached, between 50 and 70 meters. Once maximum velocity is reached, it can be maintained for only approximately 10 meters. Velocity then gradually decreases throughout the remainder of the race. Slow to fast (0 m/s→7 m/s→10 m/s→12 m/s).
Stride frequency	Stride frequency is slow at the beginning of the race, increases rapidly, and then is maintained as much as possible throughout the race.
Heel recovery	This is directly related to the height of knee lift. At the beginning of the race, the heel height and knee height are rather low. As the race continues, heel and knee height increases throughout the acceleration period. The heel height and knee height should be maintained throughout the remainder of the race.

Based on information found in the USA Track & Field Level II Sprint Curriculum.

1. Start zone. The goal of the start is to overcome inertia and get the body into an efficient position to accelerate as soon as possible. The goal is not to win the start; rather it is to place the body in position to begin a pattern of acceleration in order to ensure good distribution of effort throughout the race. The start includes the reaction to the gun and the drive from the blocks. Reaction time is the time necessary for the muscles to respond to the starting stimulus. Reaction is a conscious voluntary action under the athlete's control. It is trainable and can be improved through recognition of the correct stimulus and execution of the correct pattern of movement.

An efficient start is dictated by position in the blocks, which is determined by the strength level and body dimensions of the sprinter. The start is the zone of the race that is most influenced by absolute strength. Tremendous contractile strength is necessary both for exerting pressure against the blocks to generate the high forces to overcome inertia and for pushing against the ground in the first four to six strides where ground contact times are relatively long.

2. Acceleration zone. Acceleration is the rate of change of velocity that allows the sprinter to achieve maximum velocity in a minimum amount of time. This quality is indicated by the steepness of the speed increase. Most athletes will accelerate to their maximum speed in four to six seconds. Acceleration demands great strength and power. The skills of driving and transition are prerequisites to good acceleration. World-class male sprinters reach their maximum speed between 50 to 70 meters in a 100-meter sprint. World-class female sprinters reach their maximum speed sooner, between 40 and 60 meters. Note that slower athletes reach their maximum velocity sooner.

The first few strides of acceleration demand that the sprinter focus on pushing backward and downward against the track. In the first steps the sprinter will have a low angle of trunk flexion from horizontal. With each subsequent step, the angle of the trunk increases until the sprinter is upright. Staying low should not be taught because it will restrict hip flexion, which will hinder the increase in stride length necessary for a proper pattern of acceleration. The first step from the blocks is relatively short. Each step will progressively increase in stride length until optimal stride length is achieved. Driving refers to the action that occurs in the first three to six strides. The goal in driving is to achieve a strong and powerful extension of the legs from the hips through the ankles during each stride—triple extension. This is characterized by longer ground contact times (which decrease with each succeeding step), exaggerated arm action, and a relatively straight line through the body from head to ankle.

Transition is the gradual change in running mechanics that occurs during late acceleration into early maximum velocity. It is characterized by a higher heel recovery where the ankle of the recovery leg actually steps over the knee of the supporting leg.

3. Maximum speed zone. Maximum velocity is the most important factor for success in a 100-meter race (Bruggemann, Koszewski, and Muller 1999). Maximum speed also plays a significant role in multidirectional sports that involve moving starts. The assumption of most coaches is that the majority of sprinting by field sport athletes is mainly acceleration rather than maximum-velocity running. This is a misinterpretation of the fact that elite sprinters do not reach maximum speed until 50 meters. Because sprints in field sports are relatively short, this has led people to the erroneous conclusion that most sprints in field sports are predominantly acceleration sprints (Benton 2001). This would be true if all the sprints began from a standing position without movement. In reality, many of the sprints begin with a jogging, striding, or fast-striding start. This can have a profound effect on athletes' velocity profiles. Because the starts are moving, it is quite probable that maximum or near-maximum velocity is achieved. We know from experience that athletes who are slower achieve maximum velocity sooner. That said, the maximum-velocity, top-speed zone has been virtually ignored in training team sports. It certainly should receive attention because it offers the possibility for significant improvement.

4. Speed maintenance zone. Speed maintenance is the ability to hold the highest percentage of maximum speed through the finish. Speed maintenance and speed endurance are synonymous. This phase follows the maximum-speed phase and is closely related to it. This is highly related to sound sprint mechanics as well as alactate anaerobic capacity. It is measured by analysis of 10-meter segments in the second half of the race and comparison of the first half with the second half of the race to determine drop-off. Once the quality of maximum speed is achieved, the challenge in training is to condition sprinters to maintain that quality as long as possible. This demands high-intensity alactate anaerobic capacity and power work, which is developed over years.

For the multidirectional intermittent and transition sports, the quality of repeated sprint ability (RSA) is important to success. This is directly related to speed maintenance. This component deserves special attention in training. Seldom if ever in game situations is one all-out sprint required; rather, what is needed is the ability to repeat a sprint at angles, curves, and varied distances at highly variable time intervals.

The zone terminology is the same for the 100 meters and 200 meters; the race distribution and the length of the speed maintenance zone are the obvious differences. Race distribution will determine and direct training. To understand race distribution, think of the sprinter as a dragster with a very small fuel tank. If all the fuel is used in the first few seconds, there will be nothing in the tank to end the race. The goal of the sprinter is to carefully control the expenditure of that fuel so that as he crosses the finish line, the tank is empty. Therefore, race distribution, which is governed by the zones, is one of the most important objectives in training. The better the race distribution, the more efficient the sprinter. The more efficient the sprinter, the better the potential to achieve high speeds consistently.

Fundamental Speed Skills

The fundamental skills required for addressing the technical components in each zone are based on the PAL paradigm. PAL is an acronym for posture, arm action, and leg action. The assumption is that speed is a skill; therefore, the skill of sprinting can be taught if proper progression and principles of motor learning are applied. It has been my experience that the body has an inherent wisdom and all we need to do is put the body in key positions and let natural instincts take over. The PAL paradigm is based on those assumptions. I have used this method to teach thousands of athletes sound acceleration and sprint mechanics. All the positions are natural and allow the body to find its own correct path.

Posture is the dynamic alignment of the body. To sprint efficiently and to incorporate all muscle groups required in sprinting, the body must maintain a proper posture through all phases of the sprint. The main element of posture is the relationship of hip position relative to the torso. Posture varies with the zone of the race as well as individual strengths and weaknesses. In acceleration the posture can be described as the "triple extension" of the ankle, knee, and hip (see figure 12.1). There is an acute angle with the hips well in front of the feet and the shoulder well in front of the hips. This angle changes with each step as the feet come under the hips and the body gradually changes to an upright posture in maximal speed.

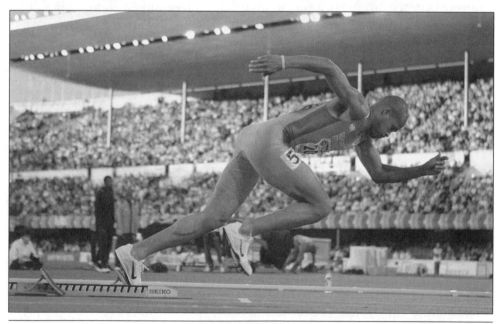

Figure 12.1 Triple extension represents the extension of the ankle, knee, and hip necessary to accelerate. The emphasis is on backside mechanics—what happens behind the body.
© Getty Images

Arm action is the second part of the PAL paradigm. There are two components to arm action: direction and amplitude. The arms should swing from the shoulders with the primary movement down and back. The arms swing to the midline of the body, but the hands do not cross the midline. The forward action of the arms is an elastic response from the stretch of the muscles of the pecs and anterior shoulder resulting from the drive back. The angle at the elbow changes from a relatively closed angle in front of the body (around 43 degrees) to an open, wide angle in excess of 110 degrees on the backstroke. The action of the arms fore and aft has been described as similar to hammering a nail. In the start and acceleration zone the arms provide a propulsive force transferring momentum to increase ground reaction forces. In maximum speed the arms serve as a balance mechanism.

The leg action is the third component of the PAL paradigm. Understanding the concept of the shin angle is the key to understanding force application during acceleration and optimizing the stride at maximum speed. The shin angle is a means of describing the relationship of the center of gravity to the ground contact point. Initially the shin angle is quite acute; this is called a positive shin angle (see figure 12.2). This allows correct use of the large muscles of the glutes extending powerfully and pushing back against the ground. A negative shin angle results in a reaching action in which the foot hits the ground in front of the shin. This results in a pulling action, which is a weak position for force application. In addition, the leg action is broken into two parts: back-side mechanics and front-side mechanics. Back side describes the leg action that occurs behind the body and front side describes the leg action that occurs in front of the body.

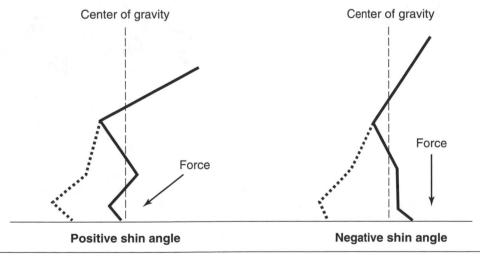

Figure 12.2   The shin angle progresses from very acute in acceleration to nearly perpendicular in absolute speed.

PAL Paradigm Acceleration Teaching Progression

The step-by-step teaching progression for acceleration applies the PAL paradigm to improve straight-ahead speed. Each drill or exercise is a step in the progression but also serves as a technique checkpoint. The following is the step-by-step teaching progression:

❶ Posture drills

Posture is the position and alignment of the body—especially the head and trunk. Posture changes with each step from the starting position through top speed. Use the following drills to improve posture:

1. **Hips tall.** Maintain relaxed shoulders. Keep the head neutral and the abdomen and butt tight.

2. **Lean or fall and walk out.** Using the tall hips position, walk out for five steps. The steps should be short and quiet. Steps that are too long will result in a slapping sound against the ground.

3. **Lean or fall and jog out.** Using the tall hips position, jog out for five steps. Each step should be slightly longer than the previous step.

4. **Fall and catch with partner.** Lean from the center *(a)*. Partner catches with the hands on the front of the shoulders *(b)*. Partner holds for five counts to let the other athlete feel the lean from the ankles and the alignment of the body.

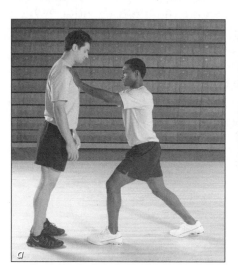 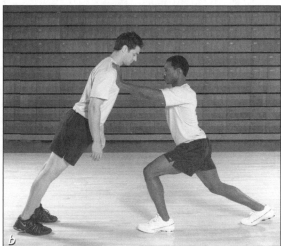

5. **Drop and go.** The partner applies support by putting both hands on the other athlete's shoulders (*a*). The partner lets the other athlete lean out as far as possible. This will teach the other athlete to initiate movement from the center as well as get the foot down to create a positive shin angle (*b*).

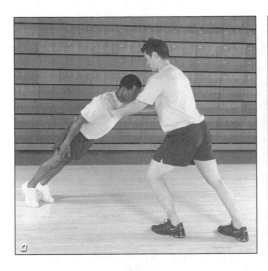
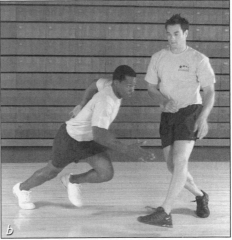

6. **Lean, fall, and run.** Put it all together into a smooth pattern of acceleration for 8 to 10 steps. Fall from the center and sprint out.

❷ Arm action exercises

Arm action is the position and amplitude of movement of the arms and hands. The arms help to produce force in acceleration and aid in balance so that force is properly applied against the ground.

1. **Giant swing—big to little.** Begin swinging the arms from the shoulders (*a*) and gradually bend the elbows (*b*) until there is a normal arm action in a sprint (*c*). Emphasize swinging from the shoulders.

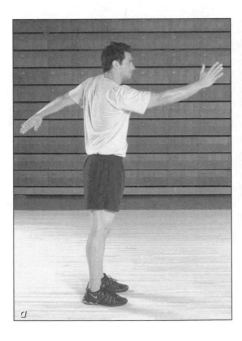
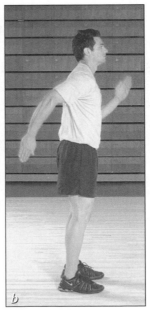
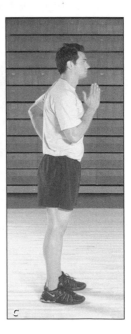

2. **Standing arm action exchange drill.** Start with one hand at chin level and the other hand in line with the opposite hip (*a*). On the command of "switch," change position of the hands with an emphasis on driving the arm down and back (*b*). See a hand in front of the chin at all times.

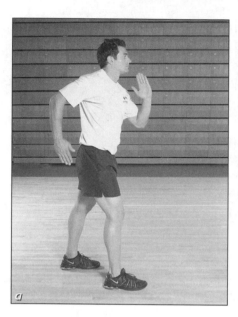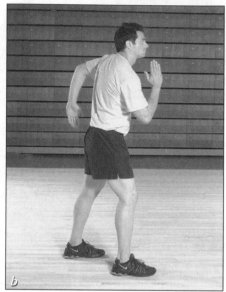

3. **Lean, fall, and run.** Focus on integration of correct arm action into the whole movement.

❸ Leg action exercises

Leg action focuses on the action of the feet, ankles, knees, and hips. The leg action in acceleration is a driving action characterized by pushing back behind the body during the initial steps. The emphasis is on back-side mechanics—what occurs behind the body. The pushing action occurs from the start through the first four to six steps. To cue the correct pattern of acceleration from the start, it is helpful to use the following verbal cues: Push . . . push . . . push . . . push . . . hips tall. This should clearly cue the push back against the ground as well as the progressive lengthening of each step and the gradual rise of the hips.

1. **Push–push drill.** Use the hips tall start position with a partner. The partner gives heavy resistance with hands on the front of the shoulders (*a*). The partner provides resistance for six steps to force triple extension of the ankles, knees, and hips (*b*).

2. **Contrast drill.** The partner gives heavy resistance for three to five steps and then gradually reduces resistance over the next three steps until there is no resistance. Then the partner releases, turns, and runs, forcing the other athlete to catch up. This will compel the other athlete to apply force correctly back against the ground and to feel the correct pattern of acceleration.

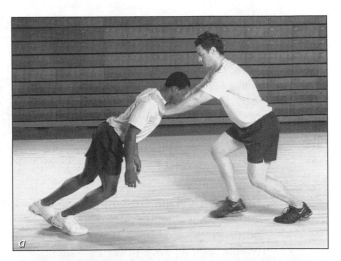

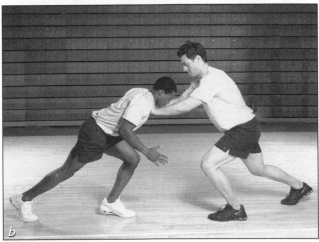

3. **Knee hugs.** Pull the knee of the free leg to the chest and hold that position until there is a full extension off the supporting (driving) leg (see figure). This will create separation between the two legs, resulting in a more efficient action of the pushing leg. Repeat the drill with the opposite leg. Actively pull the knee to the chest and then release it so that the result is an active, piston-like drive into the ground.

4. **Knee hug and go.** The partner applies support by putting both hands on the other athlete's shoulders. The other athlete initiates movement by leaning forward from the center. The partner then releases the pressure and the other athlete must get the foot down to create a positive shin angle and be in a position to run out.

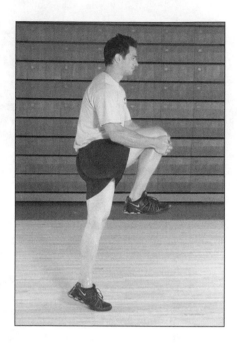

5. **Lean, fall, and run.** Always finish with the whole action to integrate all components into the whole.

PAL paradigm acceleration teaching progression adapted, by permission, from Gambetta, V., and G. Winckler. 2001. *Sport Specific Speed: The 3S System.* Sarasota, FL: Gambetta Sports Training.

MULTIDIMENSIONAL SPEED AND AGILITY

Now that the basis of speed is established, turn your attention to the other component of the 3S system: multidimensional speed and agility. To understand it, you need to know that it involves the ability to complete a given sport-specific task in the shortest time possible. It is the ability to change direction or orientation of the body based on internal and external information without significant loss of speed. It combines physical, biomechanical, and decision-making abilities. It is the maintenance of dynamic equilibrium demanded by quick acceleration and deceleration, culminating in the appropriate sport action.

Multidimensional speed and agility is a series of complex movements in the context of a specific game. The main factors influencing agility are perception, decision making, and speed in change of direction, so it is helpful to think of it as having a motor component and a cognitive component. Agility can be planned or reactive. Planned agility occurs when athletes know where they are going and can plan the movements to adapt. Reactive agility is totally unplanned; it is most applicable to actual sport situations.

Multidimensional speed and agility is the key to game speed. Not only does it have a component of performance enhancement, but it can also make a significant contribution to injury prevention. An athlete who is more agile will be able to safely get into and out of positions that would otherwise be impossible. This can be developed only through a systematic approach that has a foundation in principles of motor learning.

Multidimensional speed and agility training is speed training, not conditioning work. The principles of speed development previously discussed apply to the improvement of multidimensional speed and agility, as does the PAL paradigm. Most game situations take place in a span of 2 to 5 seconds. This work is of high neural demand and must be consistently reproduced in a climate of fatigue. This brief time does not allow an athlete to think about what to do; the action must be instinctive recall of previously rehearsed situations and movement. Start with teaching the skill. When the athletes master the skill, add reaction. When they master that, then, and only then, incorporate fatigue.

The multidirectional movement demands of field and court games dictate a reevaluation of the approach to the development of what was traditionally called agility. Surprisingly, there has been very little research analysis of the mechanics involved in changes of direction. There is some debate as to whether straight-ahead speed and change-of-direction speed are similar qualities. There are some common characteristics, but there are significant differences. Warren Young from the University of Ballarat in Australia has researched the relationship between straight-ahead speed and agility. He found that the more complex the agility task, the less the transfer of straight-ahead speed training to agility (Young, McDowell, and Scarlett 2001). For me, the link between the two is the PAL paradigm. It is still the manipulation and control of posture, arm action, and leg action in multiple directions from varied starting positions.

MDSA Training

Our understanding of game demands dictates a systematic, multifactor approach that will result in significant improvement in game speed. To effectively train agility, it is important to consider the underlying coordinative abilities and strength and how they fit in the context of the movements that occur in the game. Full development of coordinative abilities provides a repertoire of motor skills that can be adapted to deal with sport-specific movement demands. According to Drabik (1996), the coordinative abilities are as follows:

- Balance is the maintenance of the center gravity over the base of support, which is both a static and a dynamic quality.
- Kinesthetic differentiation is the ability to feel tension in movement and, based on that, to achieve the desired movement.

- Spatial orientation is the control of the body in space.
- Reaction to signals is the ability to respond quickly to auditory, visual, and kinesthetic cues.
- Sense of rhythm is the ability to match movement to time.
- Synchronization of movements in time involves unrelated limb movements done in a synchronized manner.
- Movement adequacy is the ability to choose movements appropriate to the task.

The coordinative abilities are all closely related. They are the underlying foundation for multidimensional speed and agility and the prerequisite for technical skills.

The components of multidimensional speed and agility training are combinations and applications of the coordinative abilities. Each component also represents a potential division in training to allow for systematic development of multidimensional speed and agility.

- **Body control and awareness.** This is the ability to control the body and its parts and maintain a high level of awareness of those parts in relation to the goal of the movement. This is not necessarily trained separately, but it is an integral part of most drills.

- **Recognition and reaction.** Recognition is the domain of the actual sport skills involved. It consists of the recognition of patterns and the cues that key reaction. Reaction is the ability to respond quickly to the required stimulus. It should be incorporated as soon as mastery of the movement is achieved.

- **Starting and first step.** Starting is the ability to overcome inertia. In multidirectional sports, starts can be stationary or moving or a combination, depending on the sport. The position of the first step in terms of creating a positive shin angle is crucial. The first step must be in the intended direction and the length must be relatively short to allow control for a possible change of direction. Effective starting demands a high level of concentric strength to overcome inertia. It involves the ankle, knee, and hip pushing back against the ground to propel the body in the intended direction.

- **Acceleration.** This involves attaining optimal speed as opposed to maximum speed in straight-ahead speed. There must be a situational awareness and an element of control. Game speed demands the ability to decelerate under control and reaccelerate if necessary. Mechanically, acceleration demands triple extension of the ankle, knee, and hip.

- **Footwork.** This is the relationship of hip to foot. Conceptually, agility is built from the ground up; therefore, footwork is the unifying thread in all agility work. I once heard a coach of a soccer goalkeeper tell the keeper that his feet got his hands to the ball. That is precisely why footwork is so important.

• **Change of direction.** It is initiated by shifting the center of gravity outside the base of support and then regaining control to maintain control and move in the intended direction. Change of direction involving stopping is the key to multidimensional speed and agility. It also incorporates the ability to restart when necessary, regardless of the position of the body.

• **Stopping.** Mechanically, this demands proportional bending of the ankle, knee, and hip in order to control the high eccentric loads and properly absorb shock and make the play. Not only does correct stopping have implications in terms of ability to make the play, but it also plays a primary role in injury prevention. Effective stopping demands a high level of eccentric strength.

Multidimensional speed and agility is a motor task. Since motor tasks can be learned, multidimensional speed and agility can be taught if the motor tasks involved are clearly defined and incorporated into a detailed teaching progression. Some basic concepts of motor learning underlie the training of

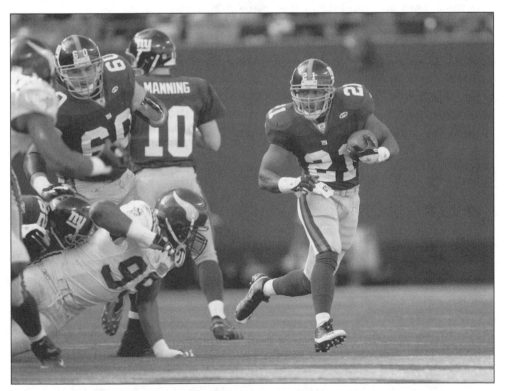

Change of direction and other applications of the coordinative abilities require a systematic approach to training multidimensional speed and agility.

multidimensional speed and agility. Understanding the difference between an open skill and a closed skill will help you design effective drills. In a closed skill, the movement is preprogrammed. An open skill occurs when the movement goal is unknown. The progression in agility training is from closed to open skills. Most agility tasks are open skills. Also, you need to differentiate between reaction and reflex. Reaction is the response to a stimulus to initiate movement. It is a conscious act that can be improved through training. Reflex, on the other hand, occurs at the subcortical (unconscious) level and cannot be trained. Practice is the actual application of all the theories. Massed practice occurs when all the skills are practiced together for a prolonged period. Massed practice has proven to be ineffective for optimal learning. Instead, distributed practice, in which a skill is practiced in small doses and recovery is allowed and then another skill is practiced at another point in the workout, is more effective.

MDSA should begin with body awareness and control in conjunction with strength training. As discussed in chapter 8, this is part of a long-term, systematic program based on fundamental movements and the subsequent refinement of those movements. Work progressively into sport skills as overall strength, body awareness, and control improve. To do this it is necessary to understand the movement patterns of the sport and the positions within the sport. Each sport has certain movement commonalities with other sports. Look for those commonalities and coach them. Each sport will also have movements that are unique to that sport. Understand those and prepare for them. Equipment will often dictate movement patterns and positions (such as the glove in baseball, the stick in field hockey and ice hockey, and the ball in rugby and football). Therefore, train and test agility, incorporating the game equipment to get a more consistent transfer to performance.

There is a school of thought that believes it is unnecessary to do any significant multidimensional speed and agility work outside the practice of the actual sport. The thought is that practicing the movements outside the sport is nonspecific work that will not transfer and that it is impossible to duplicate the intensity of the actual practice or a game. I do not share that viewpoint. If that were the case, then all that athletes would ever do is play the game and never practice. You must carefully design drills that tap into the repertoire of motor skills acquired through the movements in the specific sport. The overload should be progressive based on principles of motor learning and biomechanics and adapted to each athlete. Design a hierarchy of exercises that lead seamlessly into the sport skill:

First level: the actual movement at game speed with reaction

Second level: the movements broken into component parts and the relationship of those parts to the whole movement

Third level: coordinative abilities that underlie the skill

Progression dictates that work shift gradually as mastery is achieved from third-level activities to first-level activities. Understanding the levels means understanding the breakdown of the movements into the actual sport movements.

Use game analysis to determine the movements and game speed. Game analysis will also determine the volume of work in the actual sport, which will then determine training volumes and intensities. I have used the rule that four times the number of efforts for a particular movement in the game is high volume, three times is medium volume, and two times is low volume. Essentially you are taking the guesswork and opinion out of the process in order to be as precise as possible in the selection and prescription of exercise to produce an adaptive response that will transfer to the game. I have spent too much time drilling for the sake of drilling. Agility drills with multiple cones and sticks may look impressive, but they often have no transfer. The player will get good at the drill, but the drills do not transfer to the game. The drills should not be an end in themselves; they should be a means to an end. Time the drills whenever possible to provide feedback to the players. That goal should be efficient, effortless, flowing movement that transfers directly to the sport.

Strength Requirements

In terms of stopping and starting, multidimensional speed and agility requires reactive strength, which is the ability to quickly absorb an eccentric load and change direction to extend the leg to accelerate. Inadequate leg and core strength will limit the quality of the movement. Lack of leg strength will significantly affect the ability to train; therefore, leg strength must be developed with agility work. The forces involved in multiple planes of movement also demand a less traditional approach to the development of leg strength so that it will transfer to the movement skills. The leg strength should be unilateral. Poor core strength will also adversely affect posture, which in turn will affect control of the center of gravity.

Basic strength is a prerequisite for force production and reduction. Eccentric strength, the primary requirement in stopping effectively, is the ability to reduce force up to nine times the body weight and the ability to change direction. It also requires tremendous joint stability and control. Force must be produced and reduced in extremely short time frames; therefore, the premium is on rate of force development. This all must be done in tenths of a second on a variety of surfaces. It is developed through exercises that build up unilateral and reciprocal leg strength. Table 12.2 shows the relationship of the necessary strength qualities to the components of multidimensional speed and agility.

All these qualities must be developed concurrently, not in isolation. Note that footwork is the unifying element in the whole process. The traditional

Table 12.2 Relationship Between Strength and MDSA Components

Strength	Footwork	MDSA Component
Basic strength		Balance, body control, and awareness
Speed strength and plyometrics		Starting and acceleration Speed angles and vectors
Power endurance		Complex footwork
Maximum strength		Change of direction, stopping

approach develops strength through repetition of the movement. In theory, as athletes get stronger the movement gets better, but it does not actually work that way. The bad habits and patterns that develop because of a lack of strength result in poor movement mechanics, which are then ingrained. Remember that it is much easier to learn a new movement than to break bad habits and relearn a movement. So even though athletes were doing the drill, the transfer was negative. Incorrect repetitions can lead to the acquisition of faulty movement patterns that further impede the formation of correct skills. A more rational approach demands mastery of prerequisite fundamental movement skills that are within the strength capabilities of the athlete. As strength increases through a systematic program, the complexity of the movements can advance in conjunction with the strength and power gains. Given the large window of adaptation open to developing athletes, this can occur quite rapidly.

Reaction and Decision Making

Perhaps the biggest shortcoming in most multidimensional speed and agility work is the lack of a reaction component. In research of simple cutting tasks, Dr. Damian Farrow (2002) of the Australian Institute of Sport has shown significant differences between patterns of activation and loading at the knee on simple cutting tasks done with reaction and the same tasks done without reaction. Reaction changes everything. It can be incorporated early and often if it is part of a logical progression. Reaction should be practiced to the dominant cue demanded by the game. In addition, perception can significantly affect movement time. In planned versus reactive activities, there is a significant increase in movement time if there is uncertainty about the direction of movement. Reaction can be a response to one of the following stimuli:

Visual: tracking ability and differentiating between a narrow and a wide focus

Auditory: voice commands, cadences, and tones

Kinesthetic: pressure, pushes, bumps, and the surface of the ground

Basic movements require abrupt changes in direction in combination with rapid movement of the limbs. Ability to use these maneuvers in the game will depend on visual processing time, reaction time, perception, and anticipation. These factors are reflected in a player's on-field agility. The purpose of most agility tests is simply to measure the ability to make rapid changes in direction and position of the horizontal plane (Farrow 2002).

We must take into account that much of the emphasis in traditional MDSA has been on planned patterns of programmed drills designed to prepare for agility tests when actual performance demands unanticipated reactions to various stimuli. Research on joint loading in cutting tasks has shown a difference in joint kinematics of a cutting task with and without reaction. Decision making changes everything; therefore it is imperative to build it into MDSA training. The challenge is to do this in a meaningful way and still teach and drill correct movement patterns.

Fundamental MDSA Skills

The PAL paradigm applies to MDSA training. The PAL paradigm is a good place to start in teaching sound movement mechanics. Movement starts with bigger body parts and moves to smaller parts. The arms play a great role in balance and application of force, and the legs actually produce or reduce force. So conceptually the PAL paradigm is a logical starting point.

• **Posture.** As you know, posture is dynamic alignment of the body. As in straight-ahead speed, this is the starting point in MDSA. In many sports the posture must change rapidly. It requires constant ability to orient the center of gravity over the base to make the play and to get the center of gravity outside the base of support with control to change direction and accelerate. Head position is a key aspect of posture. Imagine the head as a bowling ball placed on your shoulders. The sheer weight demands that you pay attention to head position because it has a profound effect on balance. The head is the rudder. Orient the head in the direction of the movement. It helps an athlete to realize that the head is the weight of a bowling ball.

• **Arms.** The arms aid in overcoming inertia. They are a key in maintaining balance without compromising their role in sport skill. A big factor in arm action is the role that the implement can play in either hindering or helping with arm action. Athletes who carry an implement in one hand typically do not use that arm effectively in movement. Just increasing this awareness can significantly improve the ability to move in multiple directions.

• **Legs.** The triple extension of the ankles, knees, and hips is crucial to acceleration; bending the ankles, knees, and hips is equally important for stopping. The first step must be in the intended direction. The point of ground contact, the impulse point, must be as quick as the game situation and the surface will allow. The key to this is to not absorb any more force than is necessary. Therefore, elastic strength is a significant prerequisite in MDSA.

Change of Direction Progression

The potential complexity of MDSA demands a detailed progression. Mastery of each step is imperative before moving on to the next step. The investment of paying attention to the details of this progression will pay rich dividends in improving the quality of movement. The progression of change of direction starts with two closed-skill drills that emphasize the control of the center of gravity and the relationship of the center gravity to the base of support. Once these drills have been mastered as closed skills, then and only then should you add reaction.

❶ Wheel drill

The first drill in the progression is the wheel drill. Begin with a stationary start and then progress to a moving start if the sport dictates that. Think of all movements forward and to the side as front spokes of the wheel. All movements over the shoulder or directly back are the back spokes of the wheel. Start with the front spokes of the wheel and then move to the back spokes of the wheel. The tempo of the exercise is step out in the desired spoke of the wheel, hold the position for one count, and step back to the starting position.

Variations

One-step wheel: The goal is to work on the position, direction, and shin angle of the first step. As the name implies, this involves only one step out through each spoke of the wheel.

Three-step wheel: This emphasizes starting and accelerating and involves more movement. The pattern of the steps is right, left, right, stop or left, right, left, stop. The steps should be driving steps at game speed.

Five-step wheel: This emphasizes starting and stopping. The pattern of the steps is right, left, right, left, stop or right, left, right, left, stop. The steps should be driving steps at game speed.

❷ Oregon shift drill

The second drill is the Oregon shift drill, which puts a premium on lateral movement. This drill was devised by James Radcliffe (1999), strength and conditioning coach at the University of Oregon. Start with a 12-inch (30-centimeter) cone in each hand, with the feet shoulder-width apart and the arms extended out from the shoulders to the sides. Squat down into an athletic position by bending the ankles, knees, and hips. Place the cones on the ground at the farthest extent of the reach and then shift, or sway, to reach each cone (a). For this initial position and when the cones are placed at a wider distance (b), the movement is only a shift of the hips in the intended direction; there should be no movement up or down, only to the side. The cones are the target to touch on each step of the progression.

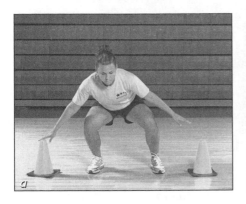 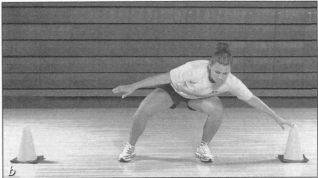

Variations

Arm span	Shift and touch the cone
Arm span plus one foot length on each side	Shift and touch the cone
Arm span and two foot lengths on each side	Shift or step and touch the cone
Arm span and three foot lengths on each side	Shift and reverse pivot and touch the cone
Arm span and three foot lengths on each side	Shift and front pivot and touch the cone
Arm span and four foot lengths on each side	Shift and shuffle slide and touch the cone

❸ Curve drills

Curves involve subtle shifts (changes) of the center of gravity over and outside the base of support. The curving movements should be trained and taught in the following sequence:

1. Lazy S: Make big, broad changes in direction.

2. Figure eight: Start big and then gradually tighten it up.

3. Circle (use hose with PVC pipe inserts to connect sections): Use circles of varying diameters.

❹ Stopping drills

The progression for teaching effective stopping is to begin at a brisk walk. Walk to flat foot from the right to the left foot or the opposite. Settling onto a flat foot slightly lowers the center of gravity, which facilitates the proportional bending of the ankle, knee, and hip to reduce force. This should result in a shin angle perpendicular to the ground. The stop should be on a flat foot in order to facilitate shock absorption by the muscles. There should be no loud slapping on the stop.

Two-foot stop

Right, left, stop

Left, right, stop

One-foot stop

Right, stop

Left, stop

The foot contacts should be quiet and rhythmic. The head and eyes should be focused on the point where you want to stop. The hips should be oriented over the feet and the shoulders over the knees. This proceeds from a walk to a run to a controlled sprint to a final step that adds reaction once the other steps have been mastered.

❺ Cutting drills

Mastery of cutting mechanics is essential for effectively changing direction. To have a systematic progression, it is necessary to define the types of cuts. Radcliffe defines them in the following way (1999). The speed cut is a cross-over pivot action: Roll off the inside foot, which is the foot nearest the intended direction of movement (*a*). The power cut involves a sit, dip, and drive: Push off the outside foot, which is the foot away from the intended direction of movement (*b*).

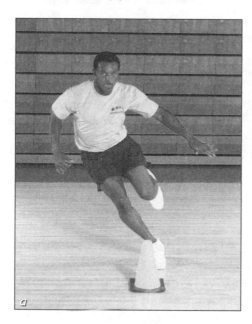 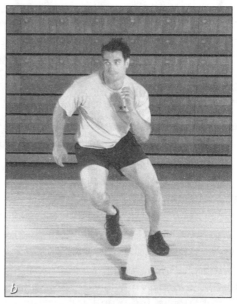

The progression goes from a walk to a run to a sprint and then adds reaction. Progress the cuts from 15 to 45 to 90 degrees. Plant the inside foot and step in the intended direction with the outside foot. Plant the outside foot and step in the intended direction with the inside foot.

SUMMARY

Of all the physical capacities, speed is probably the one that attracts the most attention. Everyone would agree that speed wins. Speed is a prized quality in athletes. Remember, though, that speed is more than the ability to sprint straight ahead. Perhaps as important to performance is multidimensional speed and agility, the component that transfers speed to performance. Both straight-ahead speed and multidimensional speed and agility can be improved significantly through a systematic program. Speed is not an isolated physical quality; it demands a high level of work capacity and outstanding strength and power. Speed involves high neural demand and demands quality, intensity, and concentration to be developed to its optimal level for each athlete.

Multiphase Performance Preparation

In the athletic development process the warm-up might just be the most important component. All athletes need a warm-up before each training session and each competition. It is an aspect of training that is very easy to take for granted because it must be a component of each training session; therefore, it tends to become quite tedious. Keep in mind that a warm-up sets the tempo for the training session. It is an integral, not separate, part of the workout. It should be thoroughly planned so that it dovetails into the actual workout. There is a real cumulative training effect from a warm-up. Think of 20 minutes minimum of warm-up each day for the duration of the training. For younger athletes, at least in the initial stages, the warm-up can be the workout. In sports with prolonged competitive seasons, the warm-up serves to maintain work capacity. So give the warm-up the attention it deserves in the whole process.

The warm-up is the bridge from normal daily activities to actual training. Too much emphasis is placed on raising core temperature and heart rate in the warm-up. The main physiological objective is neural activation, getting everything firing to prepare for the more intense work to follow in the actual workout. From a psychological perspective the warm-up should be a ritual that can function as a security point or anchor for the athletes. Try to stay away from stationary bikes and stair steppers as part of the warm-up. These machines encourage a restricted range of motion (that is, they shorten the psoas muscles), which could have negative effects on the subsequent workout.

A complete and effective warm-up should be in concert with the goal of the workout. It should be progressive in that it builds in intensity in a crescendolike manner. It must be active and dynamic, not passive and static. It is a given that a warm-up should elevate the heart rate and raise core temperature of the muscles, but the most overlooked and perhaps the most valuable aspect of the warm-up is stimulation of the nervous system. The nervous system is the command and control system of the body. It dictates the order, selection, and tempo of the tasks involved in the warm-up.

WARM-UP STAGES

Warm-up consists of multiple stages that fall into two broad categories: general warm-up and specific warm-up. The stages are not equally divided; the proportion is usually 75 to 80 percent general to 20 to 25 percent specific. The specific warm-up segment is usually the first segment of actual practice; it consists of sport-specific activities usually done at a lower intensity. The stages of warm-up are sequenced to work from the ground up and the core out. There is an emphasis on hip position, awareness, and mobility.

If multiple training sessions are planned for a day, then each warm-up after the first warm-up should be abbreviated. I have no research foundation for this, but I have observed what I call a metabolic spillover effect after the initial warm-up. Once there is an initial warm-up, the metabolic effect of that warm-up seems to linger for two to three hours and sometimes even longer in a hot, humid environment. Core muscle temperature and range of motion do not decline rapidly with the cessation of exercise, especially if there is a thorough cool-down. Therefore, if you are doing multiple training sessions in a day or you are competing in a tournament situation that calls for several matches or games in a day, the second and third warm-up do not need to be as extensive. In fact, each succeeding warm-up should be more abbreviated and more specific to the needs of each athlete. This is important in terms of conserving energy and optimizing performance. Each succeeding warm-up needs to be less extensive unless there is a period longer than four hours from the end of the previous cool-down to the beginning of the next warm-up. The toughest part of multiple warm-ups is addressing the issue of neural activation. The challenge here is not to overdo it so as to dull the nervous system.

It is also important to point out that the warm-up is very individual. If an athlete has an excitable makeup, then the warm-up does not have to be as long. The opposite is true for the mellow, more passive athlete. In team situations you need to take these individual factors into account. The key is that all the team members should be prepared for the start of the practice or game. As an athlete progresses through the career and gains more experience, the warm-up functions as a daily ritual. I remember watching Edwin Moses, two-time Olympic champion in the 400-meter hurdles, warm up. I watched him train daily for two years. His routine never varied; he did the same exercises in the same order every day, regardless of the conditions. The whole routine took 45 minutes, and when he was finished he was ready to train or compete. Competition warm-up should be different in some regards than practice warm-up. It should include most of the elements of the practice warm-up adjusted to the conditions and demands of the competition. It can serve as a tool for psychological arousal or calming as needed. Competition warm-up must be flexible so that athletes can adapt to different space requirements.

SAMPLE ACTIVE WARM-UP

The warm-up can vary in length from as short as 10 minutes for the warm-up before a second session to as long as 30 minutes. The length ultimately will be determined by the objective of the workout. The warm-up should be active but not continuous. This distinction is important. Active refers to the fact that the warm-up consists of movements that are active and dynamic, not passive exercise like static stretching. Continuous means that there are no breaks between warm-up activities. This can be used occasionally, especially on a recovery day or on a day that emphasizes work capacity and the subsequent workout is of low neural demand. The warm-up should build progressively in intensity into the workout. The emphasis is on joint mobility, not on static flexibility. Flexibility is trained as a separate unit, preferably after the workout. In a cold environment, proper clothing can greatly prolong and enhance the effect of the warm-up. After a warm-up it is helpful to towel off, hydrate well, and change into dry clothes for the actual workout. The following are the stages of active warm-up.

Active Multistage Warm-Up

❶ Progressive strides

6 to 8 strides × 50 meters

This exercise raises core temperature. These are not jogs but relaxed strides that enhance good running mechanics. The last thing you want is to have the athletes start the workout by plodding. Start at 50 percent effort and end at 70 percent effort.

❷ Leg swings

Swing forward and back

Swing side to side across the body

This exercise dynamically loosens the hip girdle.

❸ Miniband routine

Sidestep (*a*)

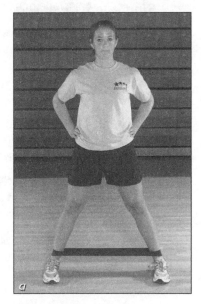

Walk forward and back (*b*)

Carioca (*c*)

Monster walk (*d*)

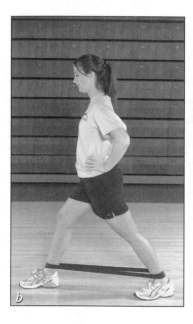 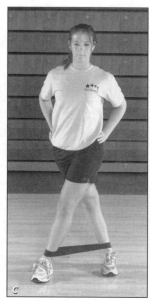 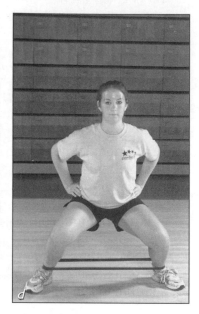

Use a 12-inch, or 30-centimeter, band above ankles. These exercises are designed to strengthen and activate the small intrinsic muscles of the hip. This segment is a key factor in prevention of low-back and groin injuries.

❹ Balance and stability exercises

Single-leg squat (hold each position for five counts)

Straight 2 × each leg

Side 2 × each leg

Rotation 2 × each leg

Balance shift

Shift and step right, shift and step left

Forward step right, forward step left

Back step right, back step left

The single-leg squat addresses static balance and the balance shift addresses dynamic balance. This segment helps with neural activation and increases body awareness.

❺ Basic core exercises

Wide rotation × 20 forward and backward

Tight rotation × 20 forward and backward

Side to side × 20 forward and backward

Figure eight × 20 forward and backward

Use a 3-kilogram medicine ball. This segment activates the core in functional positions. (See chapter 9 for more on core exercises.)

❻ Multidimensional stretch

Lunge and reach series (2 reps in each plane)

Forward (*a*)

Side (*b*)

Rotational (*c*)

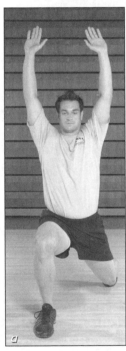 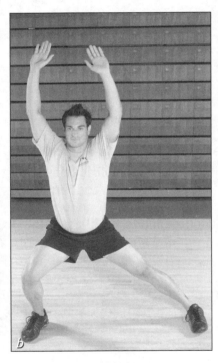 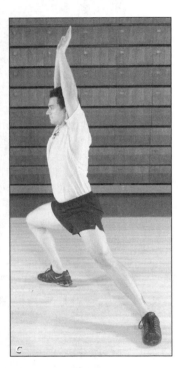

This series works through wide ranges of motion to promote mostability. In addition to reaching up, other variations include reaching out and down or across while performing the lunges.

❼ Active stretch

Psoas stretch

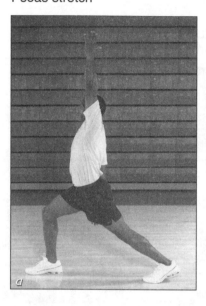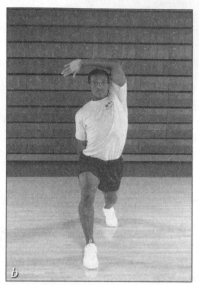

The emphasis here is on active stretching in three planes of motion for the key target areas that are needed by that person. Every person should have his or her own routines based on individual needs. Due to the increased time we spend sitting during the day, the psoas stretch is a good addition to every athlete's active stretch routine.

❽ Crawl

Jackknife crawl × 5

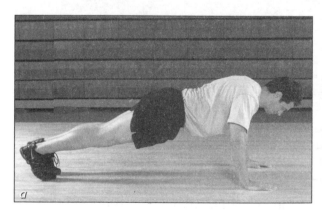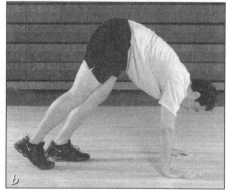

Creepy crawl × 5

This works the core and reinforces opposition.

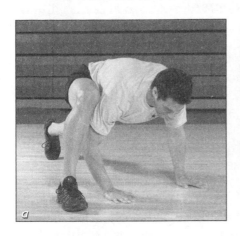

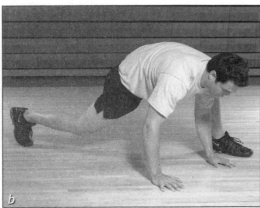

❾ Hurdle walk

Hurdle walk over

Use five hurdles. This segment addresses dynamic hip mobility.

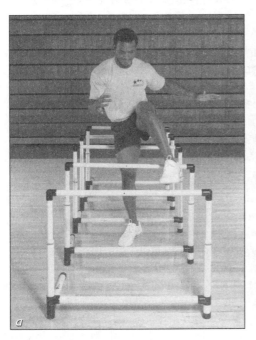

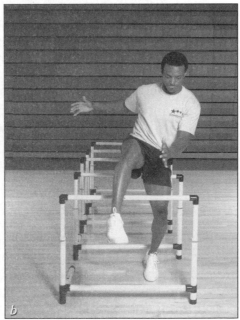

⑩ Coordination exercises

Coordination 1 (2 reps of each exercise)
Skip
Crossover skip
Side step
Carioca (low and long)
Carioca (short and quick)
Backward run
High-knee skip
High-knee skip with rotation

Coordination 2 (2 reps of each exercise)
Serpentine stride 2 × 30 yards (27.4 meters)
Crossover skip with rotation 2 × 30 yards
Angle sidestep 2 × 30 yards
Carioca quick change 2 × 30 yards
360-degree turns 2 × 30 yards (four turns)
Line touches 2 × 30 yards
Forward into backpedal 2 × 30 yards
Backpedal, turn, and go 2 × 30 yards

The coordination segment is just that: It is designed to promote coordination and body awareness. The coordination 1 module is more linear; the coordination 2 module involves more change of direction. Alternate the two based on the objective of the subsequent workout.

SUMMARY

The warm-up may be the most important part of each training session. Give as much attention to planning the warm-up as you do to the workout. A good warm-up will give the athlete a preparation routine, which can serve as a psychological anchor to performance. Warm up to play; do not play to warm up. Also remember that a warm-up is more than raising core temperature; it activates the nervous system and prepares it for the subsequent demands of the actual workout. Remember to plan the warm-up as thoroughly as the workout to ensure that the warm-up and the workout mesh and produce the optimal training effects.

Recovery and Regeneration

"**R**emember that the tour will be won off the bike." This is a statement about restoration from a member of the support staff for a Tour de France rider. After all the work is done, athletes need a sound strategy for recovering from the stress of the work to enhance adaptation or, in case of competition, come back ready for the next game, match, or stage. Mike Shannon, exercise physiologist at the U.S. Olympic training center in Chula Vista, California, calls recovery and regeneration *invisible training*. It also has been called *the hidden workout* or *the silent workout*. Recovery is something that is not as visible as running a specific sprint interval or lifting a certain weight. Yet it is just as crucial to the training process. It certainly is a process, not a one-time event. According to Kellmann (2002), "Recovery, an essential component of athletic training and a counterbalance to training and nontraining stress, is too often overlooked" (p. 3). This underscores the necessity of having a sound recovery strategy as part of the training plan.

Adaptation to training occurs during the recovery. After the work, the rest should be easy. According to Dan Benardot, "Recovery is the process the athlete goes through to return to a state of performance readiness. Recovery involves a restoration of nutrient and energy stores, a return to normal physiological function, a lessening of muscle soreness, and disappearance of the psychological symptoms (irritability, disorientation, inability to concentrate) associated with extreme fatigue" (Arnett et al. 2001).

My awareness of recovery as a formal proactive process was raised in 1994 at the post-Commonwealth Games coaching conference in Victoria, Canada. The literature on recovery up to that point came primarily from the former Eastern Bloc countries. Many of the techniques did not seem very practical to me. In addition, the information seemed flawed because of the role that systematic doping played in the overall system, most specifically as a recovery methodology. I realized that to get better and more consistent results from training, I needed to structure the recovery. Therefore, I attended two workshops on recovery and regeneration. One was presented by Angie Calder, a pioneer in the field, who at that time was the person in charge of recovery and regeneration at the Australian Institute of Sport in Canberra. The other was presented by Wynn Gimitrowski, a physical therapist and middle-distance coach from Canada. Angie and Wynn worked in a drug-free environment and developed a systematic approach to recovery that worked in an environment similar to what most of us experience. Before I attended these workshops, recovery was not a central theme in my training programs; it was something done on so-called recovery days. It was not part of the daily regimen. It was done by chance, not by design. It certainly was not a proactive process.

After assimilating the information from those workshops, I began to search for an in-depth understanding of the methodology of recovery and regeneration. This was significantly enhanced when I was able to work with Angie Calder on a daily basis at a training camp with the Australian women's Olympic softball team. This was an eye opener! We trained two or three times a day. Recovery sessions were scheduled after each training session. These consisted of hot-and-cold contrast baths, swimming pool work, and self-massage. The results were nothing short of amazing. The athletes' recovery from session to session and day to day was incredible. They did not have the degree of soreness and cumulative fatigue that I would have expected given the type of work they were doing. That experience taught me that recovery must be an integral part of every training session—not just between training sessions but also between drills and exercises.

OVERTRAINING

To better understand recovery, you need to understand overtraining. It is a process of several factors that culminate in a dramatic decline in performance and ability to train. The result is due to a failure to consider the process of training and recovery as a unified whole.

Much of the current literature and scientific understanding of recovery are spin-offs of the research on overtraining. Successful athletes must be able to push themselves, sometimes to the edge. With today's competitive climate that exists at all levels, the phenomenon of overtraining is more of a possibility than ever before.

It is impossible to improve as an athlete without a certain threshold of training stress. As athletes begin to train harder (especially younger developing athletes), the improvement is usually commensurate with the increase in training. Eventually there is a point of diminishing returns, in which increased workload will not necessarily lead to further improvement. At this juncture athletes must begin to balance the components of the program and carefully plan rest and recovery in order to realize continued improvement. Generally this will occur between the training ages of four and six and should be part of a long-term plan so that it does not come as a shock to the athletes.

Overtraining Causes

One issue for today's athlete is the frenetic pace of modern lifestyle. I recently saw it referred to as an overcommitted lifestyle. Developing athletes who are trying to balance school, relationships, work, family responsibilities, and training are very susceptible to overtraining. Professional athletes, who must produce scores as well as maintain all the outside commitments demanded by the team, agents, endorsements, and family and personal responsibilities, are prime candidates for overtraining.

There are many other causes of overtraining:

- **Abuse of toxic substances, especially alcohol.** This is especially a problem in certain sports where postgame and postpractice alcohol consumption is part of the culture of the sport.
- **Loss of weight and extreme fluctuations in weight.** This factor is common for wrestlers, gymnasts, boxers, weightlifters, and runners. The effect of constantly having to make weight to stay in a weight class or to appear a certain way to please judges can speed up the process of overtraining.
- **Lifestyle coupled with hard training.** This is especially true with students who have to stay up late every night studying.
- **Poor nutrition.** Often it involves an inadequate or inappropriate diet for the type of training. The diet can be too low in carbohydrate, too high in carbohydrate, or lacking in protein or other essential nutrients. It could also be a vegetarian or fad diet that is lacking in essential nutrients. Iron deficiency is a result of an unbalanced diet. Intraworkout nutrition, especially hydration, is often neglected.
- **Neglect of recovery.** This can be a problem both intraworkout and interworkout. Different systems of the body recover and adapt at different rates, so this must be taken into consideration.
- **Heavily biased workloads.** Workouts that continue to stress one component cause a stagnation, which results in overtraining.
- **Repetitive travel, especially across multiple time zones.** This can be especially detrimental. Jet lag and changes in eating habits during travel have profound effects on recovery.
- **Poor planning.** This involves planning of workouts, competition, and recovery.
- **Monotony in training.** Doing the same thing every day at the same time in the same sequence will eventually take a severe mental toll.
- **Too much competition.** Inadequate recovery between competitions compounds the negative effects. It is less of a problem for mature elite athletes than for developing athletes.
- **Too fast a rise in intensity or volume of training.** Too much too soon does not allow the body to adapt to the stress of training.

These variables are highly interdependent. Seldom is one of these factors the sole cause of overtraining. Kurz (2001) believes that overtraining has more to do with the sequence of work rather than the total training load.

Improper sequence leads to excessive overload by not allowing the body to adequately recover.

Overtraining Prevention

We know that overtraining is more than normal fatigue. Once an athlete is overtrained, it is a serious problem and it is difficult to reverse the symptoms. The best way to prevent overtraining is by thorough planning of training and recovery. Careful consideration needs to be given to training loads, recovery time and training modalities, and the competitive schedule. More is not better. In many sports, especially the speed and power sports, volume is not the stimulus. Intensity is the stimulus for specific adaptation. In the same vein it is imperative to remember that training is cumulative. No one session or week of training will make an athlete's career, but one session or week can break it.

Never increase volume and intensity at the same time. Always allow adequate recovery time both intraworkout and interworkout. Make sure that the diet is well balanced and appropriate to the training and sport demands. Adapt the training to the environmental conditions. If possible, control the demands of life stress. Individualize the training. No two people

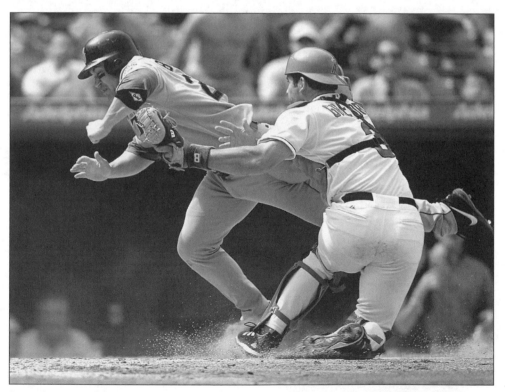

Intensity, not volume, is the key to adaptation in speed and power sports like baseball.
© Michael Zito/SportsChrome

will respond to the stress of training the same way. Closely monitor competitive stress.

Preventing overtraining involves more than rest. It often involves recognizing and changing the patterns of an addictive lifestyle. In this case the addiction is training and competition. It is closely related to self-image and self-concept. My observation is that insecure athletes with poor self-image want to do that little extra to push themselves over the edge. The same things that make an athlete successful are the same things that lead to overtraining—an insatiable desire to succeed. It is more than a willingness to work; it is actually an obsession with work.

Generally endurance athletes are more susceptible to overtraining than speed and power athletes simply because of the volume of their training. That is not to imply that speed and power athletes do not get overtrained. More often than not for speed and power athletes, their overtraining is the result of too much high-intensity work. When speed and power athletes reach an overtrained state, the effect is dramatic because of the explosive nature of their events. The events are usually measured in very small increments; therefore, any overtraining will be dramatically magnified. Also, it is less likely that team-sport athletes will be overtrained when they are training as a team. It seems that if there is positive group energy and environment, overtraining is less likely to occur. I have seen several overtrained teams but most of it was related to a tyrannical or fanatic coach who did not understand the need for recovery and variability in training.

Physiological Factors

Athletes need to learn to monitor the body and its vital signs in performance and training. Training should not be an obsession. It should be part of life.

Overtraining is a gradual process; therefore, if the early stages can be recognized, then the causative factors can be eliminated and the overtraining can be prevented. It manifests itself as trouble with technique and performance errors and is followed by performance decline. Sometimes this is so subtle that it is virtually unnoticeable.

The next stage is a gradual onset of persistent joint and muscle soreness. Things such as swimmer's shoulder, jumper's knee, or Achilles tendinitis become nagging problems. There will also be a decrease in appetite with an accompanying loss of weight. In most cases there will be increased susceptibility to colds, fevers, sore throats, and possibly allergic reactions. Tenderness, soreness, and swelling of the lymph nodes are other signs of overtraining. Lethargy away from workout is quite common. Irritability toward people and situations that do not normally cause agitation is another sign, as is profuse sweating with minimal exertion. Shortness of breath during warm-up and the feeling that the warm-up is like a workout are other signs.

The following are some physiological markers of overtraining:

- **Pulse rate.** This is not as reliable a marker of overtraining as once thought. There are too many variables that can affect heart rate, so it must be interpreted in context.

- **Intraworkout heart rate.** This is used to monitor recovery between work bouts. This can be effective for sports in which there is a high cardiovascular demand, but it is not especially valuable for speed and power athletes.

- **Morning resting heart rate.** There are many variables that affect this, which cause it to be a less reliable indicator.

- **Quality of sleep.** Restless, interrupted sleep is a good indicator. If an athlete wakes up tired, that is another sign.

- **Appetite.** Generally a loss of appetite or abnormal craving for certain foods indicate overtraining.

- **Body weight.** Unusual gains or losses and wide fluctuations in weight may indicate overtraining.

- **Joint and muscle soreness.** Muscle soreness that declines after a day or two is a normal outcome of training. Persistent soreness is not normal. Joint soreness, especially if it persists, is not good.

- **Blood measures.** This invasive measure is expensive and not readily available to most coaches and athletes.

- **Urinalysis.** This is not readily available in most situations; therefore, it is not practical.

- **Training performances.** Inability to complete a workout that an athlete previously completed with ease is an indication of overtraining.

- **Competition results.** If there is a large drop-off in performance over several competitions, it is usually a good indicator of overtraining.

Psychological Factors

One of the best ways to monitor and measure overtraining is to simply ask athletes for a subjective rating of how they feel. This, coupled with close observation by the coaches, will go a long way in preventing overtraining and assessing recovery. Remember that by the time the physiological indicators show up, the level of training is probably already approaching a state of overtraining. Psychological factors better predict the onset of overtraining than do the physiological factors. Psychological disturbances occur before the onset of the overt physiological indicators. These can be identified through psychological self-report forms, which are quite reliable. There are subjective measures—in essence, a scan of the body—that each athlete has to monitor daily. Coaches should require each athlete to keep a detailed training diary for the athlete's personal use. Training diaries consist of data on daily workouts as well as competition records. Closely monitor training and athletes' responses to training. I have found it useful, especially with students, to give them a seven-day monitoring form that asks them to report hours of sleep, meals and meal times, resting heart rate, and quality of sleep. They were required to turn this in every Monday morning on the way to class so that adjustments could be made in the subsequent week's cycle of training.

Overtraining Treatment

Complete rest for a period based on the severity of the overtrained state is usually a starting point. There is no set formula for the length of time for recovery from overtraining. Athletes are accustomed to certain levels of activity; therefore, complete rest can sometimes actually make the problem worse. Complete rest can be a negative shock to the system, so active rest, consisting of a low level of intensity, is a better alternative. This activity should be very different from normal training activities. It should be carefully designed to provide just enough stimuli for normal appetite and sleep.

Nutritional therapy, consisting of a diet higher in either protein or carbohydrate (depending on the type of overtraining), is advisable. There are various schools of thought about megadoses of vitamins; it depends on preference. Psychological counseling can be helpful, especially if it is an addictive pattern of behavior that has caused the overtraining. Psychological intervention in terms of proper goal setting and relaxation training has proved useful. Medical intervention may also be warranted, especially if an iron deficiency is present or an athlete has mononucleosis. Take all means to prevent overtraining through proper planning, because once an athlete is in an overtrained state, in most instances that competitive season is lost!

RECOVERY PLANNING

To ensure the highest-quality training and to prevent overtraining, recovery must be planned as part of the training process. I have found it beneficial to build the workout around the recovery for athletes who were finely tuned. It does no good to give athletes a workout that they could handle and then not be able to come back and do anything significant for days afterward. I realized that a key to all of this was the need to assess my athletes' "recoverability," which is how well they are able to recover from the different workloads. I did this both subjectively and objectively. No two athletes recover from the same workout the same way. In fact, athletes react individually to different types of work. I found that the recovery strategy had to match the type of fatigue. Some athletes are fast adapters and recover quite quickly; others are slow adapters and take significantly longer. This is easy to address in an individual sport, but it can present a managerial problem in a team sport. The means of assessment of recoverability is to closely monitor training and the response to training. Consider the sport classification when designing the recovery regimen. Contact and collision sports need to be treated differently because of the structural damage to muscle tissue from contact. The same is true of impact sports such as in the jumps in track and field, where there is heavy eccentric loading.

Recovery is the process needed for repairing damage caused by either training or competition. Recovery is an interindividual and intraindividual, multilevel (e.g., psychological, physiological, social) process for the reestablishment of performance abilities. Recovery includes an action-oriented component. Self-initiated activities can optimize conditioning and build up and refill personal resources and buffers (Kellmann 2002).

Recovery is a series of planned actions to bring athletes back to baseline. Activities or external means help athletes physically or psychologically overcome the rigors of hard training. Regeneration is an active process consisting of a planned training unit to help the body recover from training and to return to previous performance levels through removal of mental and physical fatigue caused by training and competition efforts. The recovery must be part of the training plan from the earliest stages of development. Recovery must be taught by making athletes more aware of reading the body and understanding how they adapt to training. It is quite a personal process that athletes must "own" in order to ensure progressive adaptation. Without recovery, the adaptation to training cannot take place.

Rest is time off with no training at all. This is a poor alternative for athletes. The body is accustomed to a certain level of activity. When that is taken away, it is a shock to the body. Complete rest interferes with appetite, sleep, and general mood state and makes the return to training more difficult. Athletes coming off a day or longer of complete rest tend to be flat rather than restored. A much more viable alternative is active rest. In active rest the muscles work, but nerves rest. It is time off from the regular activities of training. "Active" refers to other sport activities. For example, basketball players will play a game of pickup soccer or swimmers may go for a bike ride. It is absence from abuse, not absence from activity; but it still gives athletes the stimulus activity that does not compromise the system.

Recovery Objectives

The global objectives of recovery and regeneration and the general strategies for addressing them are universal. The following strategies and recommendations should serve as a guide for designing a good recovery program:

- **Restore glycogen levels.** Without a doubt, this is the primary nutritional goal of the restoration process. Failure to restore glycogen levels has profound negative implications, even to the next workout on the same day. The goal of recovery is to get glycogen levels to preexercise levels. To be effective, carbohydrate (CHO) should be taken within a two-hour window after exercise. Low glycogen will result in fatigue, dizziness, light-headedness, sleeplessness, and muscle soreness. The guidelines for replenishment of glycogen levels are 1 gram of carbohydrate per kilogram of body weight per hour for the first two hours postexercise and 1.2 grams of carbohydrate per kilogram of body weight per hour in 15- to 30-minute intervals for up to four hours postexercise.

- **Minimize the breakdown of muscle.** This is a cumulative process. Seldom can one workout cause this. The stress of several hard workouts or a very demanding competition, especially hard endurance sessions or heavy lifting sessions, puts the body in a catabolic state in which tissue is broken down. To recover, the body must repair this damaged tissue by shifting to an anabolic (muscle-building) state. The guidelines for minimizing the catabolic effect of training are to follow the protocol for carbohydrate but use a protein-to-carbohydrate ratio of 1 to 4. Research has shown that 6 grams of protein will accelerate protein synthesis after exercise.

- **Restore depleted electrolytes.** This is an ongoing process that must be addressed both intra- and interworkout. It is imperative that athletes have a well-planned strategy to address this. According to Maughan, "Electrolyte replacement is crucial. Salts act like a sponge, holding in fluid in the body. If you drink a large volume of plain water, the body thinks it is overhydrated because the water dilutes the concentrations of sodium and other dissolved substances in the blood. This switches off thirst and switches on the kidneys to increase urine output. Sodium is the most important electrolyte as it is the one lost in sweat in the greatest amounts, and that's why it is added to sports drinks" (Arnett et al. 2001). Replacement of essential electrolytes such as sodium, magnesium, potassium, chloride, and calcium can prevent heat illness, nausea, confusion, headaches, sleeplessness, postexercise fatigue, muscle soreness, and gastrointestinal distress. Athletes need to avoid colas, coffee, tea, and alcohol because these drinks have a diuretic effect that will delay the rehydration process.

- **Hydrate and rehydrate.** This is the easiest aspect of recovery to implement, but perhaps because it is so easy it is often forgotten until athletes are in a distressed state. It is a factor anywhere athletes train, not just in hot, humid environments. Hydration will stabilize the blood volume and prevent muscle cramping. The guidelines for fluid replacement are as follows: Athletes should weigh in before and after training to estimate sweat loss. Each kilogram (2.2 pounds) of weight loss is equal to one liter of sweat loss.

To rehydrate after training, drink 1.5 times the calculated volume of sweat loss. Use a commercially available drink that combines rapid absorption rates (hypotonic characteristics) with adequate amounts of carbohydrate and electrolytes.

• **Offset the effects of free radicals.** Free radicals are caused by pollution, chemicals, food additives, stress, and the combustion of energy. Athletes in sports with higher cardiorespiratory demands should be especially aware of the production of free radicals. Free radicals have the potential to kill healthy cells, prematurely age them, and alter their DNA. They can break down healthy cells, which can lead to a variety of health problems. Production of free radicals can be reversed with antioxidant nutrients such as vitamins C and E and beta-carotene and the minerals selenium and zinc.

• **Reduce inflammation.** The stress of training produces microtears and swelling in muscle tissue. Inflammation is a natural protective mechanism of the body to heal and stimulate blood flow to the damaged tissue. There must be a balance between allowing the body's natural inflammatory response to take place and minimizing swelling that could inhibit training in subsequent training sessions. The best way to reduce inflammation and stimulate blood flow is gentle movement combined with ice after cessation of exercise.

• **Reduce muscle soreness.** Muscle soreness is the natural result of training. Delayed-onset muscle soreness (DOMS) is a well-established phenomenon. With DOMS, athletes are more sore the second and third day postexercise. The steps to control DOMS are a systematic cool-down that stimulates blood flow to the targeted muscles, gentle rhythmic exercise, and static stretching. Gentle exercise in a swimming pool is very effective. Postexercise massage will also increase blood flow in the muscles but should not be used after every session of exercise. Another method involves a shower followed by a spa (39 to 40 degrees Celsius, or 102 to 104 degrees Fahrenheit) for three minutes and then a cold shower or a plunge into a cold pool (10 to 15 degrees Celsius, or 50 to 59 degrees Fahrenheit) for 30 to 60 seconds. Spas should be used only if athletes are healthy and have no new soft-tissue injuries. Athletes should also not stay in a spa for more than five minutes because they are likely to have a large drop in blood pressure (Calder 1996).

• **Boost the immune system.** Systematic high-level training will severely stress the body's immune system. This must be addressed by moderating lifestyle and through proper nutrition. It is recommended to supplement with vitamin C to enhance the immune system.

• **Acquire adequate sleep.** Get at least 8 hours of continuous sleep every night. Rest more if traveling across time zones and allow sufficient time between training sessions for recovery. If it is determined that somewhat less than the recommended 8 hours of sleep is being achieved, a "sleep debt" is incurred. If sleep debts occur, then steps should be taken to repay the sleep debt. Athletes can make up sleep debt by going to bed earlier each night for an extended period. If schedule permits, they can take a 30- to 60-minute nap during the day.

There are some basic guidelines for restoration depending on the timing in relation to the workout (table 14.1). Within the workout, allow adequate rest between exercises and the various types of work. This rest should be active in nature. A major recovery consideration intraworkout is proper nutrition. During the workout this should consist of fluid replacement and carbohydrate replacement, preferably combined. Shaking and self-massage can be effective recovery tools between exercises in a workout, especially in a training-camp environment and also with elite athletes who are doing multiple workouts within a day. Between morning and evening workouts, apply recovery methods immediately at the conclusion of the first workout. Between days, employ the recovery methods six to nine hours after the workout or competition. If the workout or competition finishes late, then start the recovery procedures in the morning after rising.

Table 14.1   Basic Guidelines for Restoration

Restoration methods during training	Rhythmic structure of training Dynamics of the rest intervals
Relaxed, free, rhythmic exercise as active rest	Activating self-massage Relaxation and stretching
Restoration methods after training	Light, free exercise Relaxation and stretching Walking Playing games
Physiotherapy	Massage Relaxing baths Sauna Hydrotherapy
Medical and biological methods of restoration	Nutrition Rhythm of meals and additional meals Vitamins and minerals
Mental training methods of restoration	Autogenic training Concentration and relaxation training

Monitoring Training

Training is a repeating (rollover) process consisting of four steps: assessment, planning, implementation, and monitoring. Monitoring this process is essential to making the training meaningful and keeping it on track. The most effective training programs that I have seen and implemented are those that have a built-in monitoring system. It does not have to be anything elaborate or scientific. Whatever it is, it just needs to be used consistently. Monitoring increases training effectiveness. The more consistent the monitoring, the more meaningful the information will be. Monitoring training allows you to reconcile what was planned for training and what was achieved. It is very specific to the sport, the performance level of the athlete, the age of the athlete, and the gender. Once a system of monitoring has been implemented, the information gathered must be straightforward and simple so that it can be easily interpreted and modifications can be made easily as needed.

The goal of training is the long-term adaptation of the cumulative training effect. You must monitor each of these effects in order to assess the program of training. Monitoring training will allow you to maintain control of the training process and ensure a proactive adaptive response. Planning the training and implementing the training are only two prongs of a three-pronged attack. Monitoring the training is the third.

Be specific. It is more than just gathering information; it is gathering information you can use. Jan Olbrecht, in his book *The Science of Winning* (2000, p. 225), gives the following analogy: "Testing a swimmer on a bicycle or treadmill in order to obtain the right information for water training is like taking temperature with a barometer; both have to do with the weather but measure something quite different." The message is clear: Monitor the training quality for which you hope to achieve adaptation. The question, then, is what should be monitored. The answer is to monitor those components of training that are the focus of that particular training period. It is not possible to monitor too much. You must look at the factors of training stress as well as total life stress factors. Monitoring should be both subjective and objective where possible. Monitor what is practical. It is different for team sports and individual sports. Remember that a team is a collection of individuals. Know what you want to do with the information you gather. Decide how training monitoring will help you.

During certain training periods where particular qualities are emphasized, other qualities should be repressed. For example, during a heavy maximal-strength block of training, explosive power and maximal speed will tend to be inhibited. This must be monitored. Perhaps the simplest training indices to look at throughout the training year that can give good objective feedback is a simple jump test protocol consisting of squat jump, countermovement jump, repetitive jump, and stiffness jump tests. These tests can be easily administered as part of training without detracting from the athletes' performance. They monitor the state of the nervous system. A one-shot battery of these tests will establish a baseline, but remember that there is a learning curve. Performance on these tests will improve with practice. This must be taken into account when establishing a baseline. These tests should be administered frequently throughout training in order to monitor training status of strength, elastic strength, and repetitive power. I want to emphasize that the comparison must be intraindividual and must be looked at serially over time.

A preworkout assessment can be useful in anticipating problems in training. It uses a 10-point scale graded from 1 ("I feel great") to 10 ("I feel absolutely awful"). I use this in comparison with the postpractice training demand rating to see if there is a relationship. My feeling is that this will give me feedback on the residual effect of the prior training session and a window into life stress. Another aspect of the training demand rating scale is that as a coach I will project what I think the training demand of a particular workout should be and I will compare that with the actual training demand as reported by the athlete. The two numbers should be fairly close. If there is a wide divergence, then I really need to reassess the process. The key to this is honest feedback from athletes. They are active participants in the process. I stress that training is not something you do *to* the athlete; it is something you do *with* the athlete. The training demand rating scale will make training work for each athlete.

Perhaps the simplest and most effective means of monitoring training is a detailed training log. The log is an athlete's personal monitoring tool. It should represent the athlete's input about responses to training. Each log, regardless of the sport or person, should contain certain basic information. The log should monitor factors outside of training: sleep, diet, and other stressors that can have an effect on training (see figure 14.1). The coach's training log should be as detailed as possible and still practical in order to isolate variables to identify possible patterns. It should incorporate the following: evaluation of planned work versus work completed, rating of the athlete's response to the work, and a breakdown of the duration of each training component.

The rating of perceived exertion scale (Borg 1998) is another valuable tool, and it can be easily adapted for use in a team as well as an individual sport. It can be used in rating training demand on individual components of the workout or for the workout as a whole. It really depends on how detailed you want to get. Regardless of how you apply it, it provides reliable feedback on the stress of training in healthy exercisers. Perceived exertion is certainly not a new concept. It originated with Gunnar Borg, a Swedish

Figure 14.1
ATHLETE'S LOG

Day _____   Date _____

Time of training _____   Hours of sleep _____

Weather (include temperature, humidity, and wind conditions)

_____

_____

Duration of the session (rounded to the nearest quarter hour) _____

Energy rating before workout (circle one):

    1   2   3   4   5   6   7   8   9   10

The Workout

Theme _____

Goal _____

Exercises:

Sets _____   Reps _____

Times _____   Interval _____

Intensity _____

Comments:

_____

_____

_____

_____

Fatigue index—posttraining (circle one):

    1   2   3   4   5   6   7   8   9   10

From V. Gambetta, 2007, *Athletic development: The art & science of functional sports conditioning*, (Champaign, IL: Human Kinetics).

exercise scientist, who designed an RPE scale for use in monitoring training stress in cardiac rehabilitation (see figure 14.2). Conceptually, athletes simply rate how hard they think they are working by assigning a number to the sensation of their effort.

For simplicity and ease of use, many coaches use a 10-point scale that has proven to be effective in the athlete population. Athletes must first be educated on the effort relative to the assigned numerical value. It must be fine-tuned for each athlete in order to provide reliable feedback on training stress. I use such a scale by having the athlete, at the conclusion of the workout, state out loud or in writing the effort of the workout. I have found it useful once I orient the athletes to the scale to allow them to develop their own verbal descriptors for the various points on the scale. This personalizes the process, which makes the information that much more meaningful.

6	No exertion at all
7	
8	Extremely light
9	Very light
10	
11	Light
12	
13	Somewhat hard
14	
15	Hard (heavy)
16	
17	Very hard
18	
19	Extremely hard
20	Maximal exertion

Borg RPE scale
© Gunnar Borg, 1970, 1985, 1994, 1998

Figure 14.2 Borg RPE scale.

Reprinted, by permission, from G. Borg, 1998, *Borg's Perceived Exertion and Pain Scales* (Champaign, IL: Human Kinetics), 47.
© Gunnar Borg, 1970, 1985, 1994, 1998

Monitoring will also help you assess how the performance was achieved. Two athletes can do the same workout, achieve the same results, and have opposite adaptive responses. One may have to tap deep into the adaptive reserve to achieve the result and the other may require much less effort. That is why it is so important to have additional means of monitoring training. Also monitor readiness for the workout and monitor indices of adaptation.

SUMMARY

After the work, the rest should be easy. The rest and recovery period is the time when training adaptation occurs. Therefore, this element of training must receive equal emphasis with all the components of work if training is to achieve the desired effect. It must be planned so that is it proactive, not reactive. Without proper rest and recovery, optimal training adaptation will not occur. Anyone can work, but allowing the work to take effect demands a good recovery plan.

The Future of Functional Conditioning

In the 21st century, the field of athletic development is still in its infancy. The opportunities to move forward, innovate, and define the field certainly exist. The essential question is whether the coaches, and for that matter all involved, embrace change and continue to move ahead or stay mired in the status quo. Tom Kelley, in *The Art of Innovation* (2001), states the dilemma: "No one gets ahead by copying the status quo" (p. 278). Moving forward and raising the level of training with the next generation of athletes will require a significant paradigm shift—a move away from the Newtonian, linear, reductionism approach that has gotten you to this point but will hold you back from making progress. Advances in science in the 20th century logically led us to a quantum approach to training, which focuses on relationships and connections. Coaching is no more than learning to take advantage of these constantly changing relationships. Using this approach, training literally becomes a dance of discovery. It requires the coach to be more involved in monitoring all aspects of training. It is a significant departure from focusing on the parts and assuming that the parts will come together in a sensible, usable whole. Constantly look for critical connections that will allow the body to adapt to the stress of training. The body is a fully integrated system; to optimize the performance of this system you must take a systems approach to training.

Change and growth are not always comfortable. Accomplishing growth demands a shift in the education and training of coaches. Coaches need to be big-picture thinkers. They cannot get caught up in minutiae and anatomical curiosities. Education needs to stress the importance of context and relationships, not isolated facts. The best coaches that I have known are consummate generalists. They are not great coaches by chance. They understand all the complex relationships that the human body possesses when trying to achieve high-level athletic performance. If this was true in the past with great coaches like Bowerman, Counsilman, and Vigil, it is even truer today. The trend today is toward specialization and further compartmentalization, which is a big mistake. For example, you can be a speed coach, but it is impossible to coach speed without an in-depth understanding of the other physical qualities. The reason given for specialization is the explosion of information and the need to apply it. This should not be a factor. Being a great coach demands understanding the big picture and the ability to enhance relationships and connections. (Remember the body constants from chapter 2.) Humans are not training machines that can be programmed; you cannot take out a part and replace it with a new one. The body is a living system that is constantly changing and adapting.

The consensus is that today's athletes are different. To reach this generation of athletes, you need to understand why they are different and what you must do to reach them. The athletes today have many conveniences available to them that did not exist 30 years ago. Turning back the clock is not an option, so you must learn to address the changes and adapt accordingly. The athletes of today simply are not as active outside of training and participation in their chosen sports; they are the products of a sedentary spectator society. Consequently you must account for that in the training environment. Young beginners do not have a base of general fitness and movement skills. Generally, elites have specialized earlier, and consequently there are more injuries that could be prevented by a broader base of preparation. Despite this, athletic performances are off the spectrum compared to those of 30 years ago, so something must be right. There is no doubt that the monetary and tangible rewards are significantly greater now than ever before. This certainly changes the approach to training. Sport does not live outside of society, so coaches need to place sport in the context of society. Be an anthropologist: Pretend you are sent into a foreign, even hostile, culture, take a step back, and try to understand the behavior you are seeing. I must admit that the current generation of athletes sometimes baffles me with their behavior, but when you put it in the context of society as a whole, it is easier to understand. As a coach, you should never compromise your core beliefs, but you must understand where the athletes are coming from. For many athletes today, training and excelling in a sport are more important for coaches than for the athletes. Coaches have much more on their plate and many other avenues to success available to them. Today's athletes must be told why they are doing what they are doing. You have to be better than ever at communicating and selling what you are doing.

It certainly is an information-driven society, but information is not always equated with knowledge. Today we have unlimited sources of information, but it is up to us to put it in a context framed by our beliefs, experience, and education to transform that information into knowledge. This is not always easy for coaches. Athletes and parents access the same information as the coaches do. Gary Winckler, women's track and field coach at the University of Illinois, sums it up quite well: "Get them off the Internet and stop them from looking for shortcuts. The human body does not adapt any faster than it did 30 years ago, so why should we expect performance gains to be accomplished faster today? A new challenge I face today that I did not face as a coach 10 years ago is helping athletes get the 'noise' out of their lives and learn to focus on the training process." The explosion of information is "noise." They, the athletes, do not have the background to differentiate good information from fallacious information. This makes it even more imperative that the coach stay on the cutting edge in terms of knowledge. The information that is acquired needs to be put in context. A good way to cross-check information and stimulate new ideas is to form a local coaches' colloquium or network to share knowledge. Include ATCs, physical therapists, and doctors in this network. This does not have to be formal. Meet once a month with a suggested topic for each session. In a group situation you quickly realize that there are commonalities both in terms of problems and solutions. If everyone agrees to share ideas and information and not let egos interfere, it's a great way to keep learning.

Frank Dick, Britain's chief coach during the golden age of athletics in the 1980s, expressed today's dilemma in coaching: "Somewhere in the last 10 years or so we have lost our place as coaches; somebody, somewhere has decided coaching cannot be respected in the way that it used to be. If this is not addressed quickly then who is going to lead the athletes? Don't tell me the scientists can. Science has never led sport. It is coaches that lead the process. As Winston Churchill said, scientists should be on tap but never on top." Coaching is always a delicate balance of art and science. The art cannot be taught, but it is something that can be acquired through experience. A coach must use science and be scientific without trying to be scientists. I am not sure that coaches today are well prepared in the science of teaching. In the past the majority of coaches were affiliated with the schools as teachers, either in the classroom or in physical education, so they had a good background in pedagogy. Coaching and teaching are synonymous. Coaches need better training as teachers. Some very good programs exist, such as the USA Track & Field Coaching Education program. We need more programs like that to educate and raise the standard of coaching.

Athletes today start specializing in a chosen sport younger than ever before. Because of this young athletes do not acquire the broad base of fundamental movement skills and they are "taught" specific sport skills that are not commensurate with their physical, cognitive, and emotional maturation levels. I have alluded to this at several places in the book. This is an alarming trend that has many long-term consequences. Certainly in most cases the young athletes have the specific sport skill and physical capabilities to excel, but what about for the long term? The early specialization can result in long-term stagnation. In reality, the ones who would have made it anyway do so because they matured early or just simply were more talented. At the other end of the spectrum there is greater incentive to compete longer because of the monetary rewards that are available in the later years of an athlete's career. There is no simple solution to this. Intuitively we certainly know that the human cost is high. We always hear about those who made it, but what about the many who are cast by the wayside? The goal in youth sport should be to provide a good experience by teaching fundamentals and the rules, not by trying to identify the next National

League MVP or Cy Young Award winner. Give them the opportunity to be kids. Play and playfulness are great qualities that allow young athletes to discover their bodies and explore the limits of their movements. They need to have room to grow and discover through movement. Bring in the play element early and keep it there!

A positive trend is the continued opportunities for women to compete in sport. Unfortunately the training and preparation have not kept pace with the opportunities to compete. Biologically and socioculturally, women are different from men. These differences must be accounted for in training and preparation. Women are certainly more susceptible to certain injuries, specifically ACL tears; this demands that prevention programs be incorporated in daily training. To do otherwise would be remiss. There is still much misunderstanding about the role of strength training with female athletes. Some athletes and coaches just do not recognize its importance. Culturally in many circles it is not acceptable for women to be muscular and fit. For female athletes to receive proper training, these barriers need to be broken down.

There is no doubt about the need for more qualified women in coaching. The time commitment and lifestyle dissuade many women because of family obligations and the general sociocultural attitude toward women in coaching. It was interesting to see the 2005 women's NCAA basketball final with the final two teams coached by women for the first time. Why did it take so long? Women need positive role models as coaches. They need to be mentored. The typical approach has been for outstanding female athletes to go into coaching upon retirement. This approach sets them up for failure. Ability to excel in a sport seldom equates with coaching success. They need to be educated and mentored so that they can truly coach.

There is no need to make things complex. The interplay between all the training variables will take care of the complexity. A few simple drills or exercises properly combined can have a significant training effect. As a coach, you need to think of yourself as a tour guide, carefully leading athletes to their destination without being overbearing, but not allowing them to get lost. To accomplish this, you must constantly look for commonalities and familiar patterns and take advantage of the relationships that will appear. Learn to foster those relationships.

Possibly the most negative cloud growing on the horizon is the specter of performance-enhancing drugs. It shouldn't be surprising that a society that thrives on instant gratification would have a problem with drugs. Performance-enhancing drugs are a huge problem at every level of sport today. Anyone who thinks otherwise is incredibly naïve. To me there is a clear division between those who do and those who don't. This extends to coaches and therapists. I made the choice years ago to not allow my athletes to use drugs. I know coaches and administrators who have the attitude that if they do not know about it, then there is no problem. Face the facts: Some of the athletic icons of our society are under great suspicion. I do know that testing is not the answer. There are people all over the United States hanging around gyms who know more about drugs and how to beat the tests than the people who are doing the testing. Save the money. Education is the answer, but what kind of education? Focus on educating the coaches to understand there are no shortcuts. The scare stories about shrunken testicles do not work; youngsters and seasoned pros just think it won't happen to them. The answer is pretty idealistic: Let's make it an ethical issue. It is flat-out cheating. Those athletes who are doping and those coaches who condone it are living a lie. Sure, they are getting scholarships and some are making millions—so what? At the end of the day you have to live with yourself. Doping is wrong. It degrades sport and the value of competition. The athletes and coaches who are working hard and smart must stand up to stop this alarming trend.

There is no doubt that advances in technology and applied sport science will have significantly more effect on the new generation of coaches. The biggest dilemma that coaches face in incorporating technology and advances in sport science is the time to learn the technology or the new methodology. The technology is there now, but is it practical? Coaches need to know what to do with the additional information. GPS monitoring of movement patterns in a game and a comparison to practice certainly offer great potential to make training more specific to the demands of the sport and the position. Breaking down this information could require up to two more hours a week. Where can coaches find the time? This is perhaps the biggest obstacle that coaches face in innovation and change: how to better use the time available as well as stay on the cutting edge. Author Gail Sheehy states it quite succinctly: "If we don't change, we don't grow. If we don't grow, we aren't really living."

As I see the enthusiasm and passion of the young people getting into the field, I think the future is bright. Those of us who have been in the field for a while must provide guidance and leadership for the next generation. That is our responsibility. The possibilities in the field are unlimited. I hope some of the insights and experiences I have related in this book will help those who are starting out to get on the functional path and follow it to its successful conclusion.

References

Anderson, O. 2000. *Running Research News* 16 (7): 1-4.

Arnett, B., D. Bernadot, R. Maughan, B. Steuerwald, and F. Tedeschi. 2001. Speeding recovery from exercise. *Gatorade Sports Science Institute Roundtable* 12 (46): 4.

Baker, D. 1995. Selecting the appropriate exercises and loads for speed-strength development. *Strength and Conditioning Coach* 3 (2): 8-16.

Benton, D. 2001. Sprint running needs of field sport athletes: A new perspective. *Sports Coach* 24 (2): 12-14.

Benton, D., and W. Young. 2001. The effects of static and dynamic stretching on block start performance. Unpublished study.

Billat, V.L., J. Slawinksi, V. Bocquet, P. Chassaing, A. Demarle, and J.P. Koralsztein. 2001. Very short (15 s-15 s) interval-training around the critical velocity allows middle-aged runners to maintain $\dot{V}O_2$max for 14 minutes. *International Journal of Sports Medicine* 22: 201-208.

Billat, V.L., J. Slawinski, V. Bocquet, A. Demarle, L. Lafitte, P. Chassaing, and J.P. Koralsztein. 2000. Intermittent runs at the velocity associated with maximal oxygen uptake enables subjects to remain at maximal oxygen uptake for a longer time than intense but submaximal runs. *European Journal of Applied Physiology* 81 (3): 188-196.

Borg, G. 1998. *Borg's perceived exertion and pain scales*. Champaign, IL: Human Kinetics.

Bruggemann, G.P., D. Koszewski, and H. Muller. 1999. *Biomechanical research project Athens 1997: Final report.* International Athletics Foundation. Oxford, UK: Meyer & Meyer.

Calder, A. 1996. Unpublished paper on recovery. Canberra: Australian Institute of Sport.

Coyle, D. 2005. *Lance Armstrong's war.* New York: Harper Collins.

Dominquez, R.H., and R.S. Gajda. 1982. *Total body training.* New York: Warner.

Drabik, J. 1996. *Children and sports training.* Island Pond, VT: Stadion.

Enoka, R.M. 1994. *Neuromechanical basis of kinesiology.* 2nd ed. Champaign, IL: Human Kinetics.

Farrow, D. 2002. Contribution of perceptual information to agility: The skill of agility. Presentation at Australian Institute of Sport, Canberra Sprint and Agility Testing Workshop.

Fleck, S.J., and W.J. Kraemer. 1997. *Designing resistance training programs.* 2nd ed. Champaign, IL: Human Kinetics.

Fox, E.L., and D.K. Mathews. 1974. *Interval training: Conditioning for sports and general fitness.* Philadelphia: Saunders.

Gabbard, C., E. Leblanc, and S. Lowy. 1987. *Physical education for children: Building the foundation.* Englewood Cliffs, NJ: Prentice-Hall.

Gladden, L.B. 2004. Lactate metabolism: A new paradigm for the third millennium. *Journal of Physiology* 58 (1): 5-30.

Godfrey, R.J., Z. Madgwick, and G.P. Whyte. 2003. The exercise-induced growth hormone response in athletes. *Sports Medicine* 33 (8): 599-613.

Hannaford, C. 1995. *Smart moves: Why learning is not all in your head.* Arlington, VA: Great Ocean.

Hawley, J., and L. Burke. 1998. *Peak performance: Training and nutritional strategies for sport.* St. Leonards, NSW: Allen & Unwin.

Hemery, D. 1976. *Another hurdle.* London: Heinemann.

Ives, J.C., and G.A. Shelley. 2003. Psychophysics in functional strength and training: Review and implementation framework. *Journal of Strength and Conditioning Research.* 17 (1): 177-186.

Johnson, G. 1996. *Fire in the mind.* New York: Vintage.

Jones, N.L. 1986. *Human muscle power.* Champaign, IL: Human Kinetics.

Kelley, T. 2001. *The art of innovation: Lessons in creativity from IDEO, America's Leading Design Firm.* New York: Doubleday.

Kellmann, M., ed. 2002. *Enhancing recovery: Preventing underperformance in athletes.* Champaign, IL: Human Kinetics.

King, I. 2000. *How to write strength training programs.* 2nd ed. Toowong, Australia: King Sports.

Kraemer, W.J., and K. Häkkinen, eds. 2002. *Strength training for sport.* London: Blackwell.

Kraemer, W.J., and N.A. Ratamess. 2003. Endocrine responses and adaptation to strength and power training. In *Strength and power in sport.* 2nd ed. Ed. P.V. Komi. London: Blackwell.

Kreighbaum, E., and K.M. Barthels. 1995. *Biomechanics: A qualitative approach for studying human movement.* 4th ed. Boston: Allyn and Bacon.

Kurz, T. 1994. *Stretching scientifically: A guide to flexibility training.* 3rd ed. Island Pond, VT: Stadion.

Kurz, T. 2001. *Science of sports training.* 2nd ed. Island Pont, VT: Stadion.

LaStayo, P.C., J.M. Woolf, M.D. Lewek, L. Snyder-Mackler, T. Reich, and S.L. Lindstedt. 2003. Eccentric muscle contractions: Their contribution to injury, prevention, rehabilitation, and sport. *Journal of Orthopaedic & Sports Physical Therapy* 33 (10): 557-571.

Lieber, R.L. 2002. *Skeletal muscle structure, function and plasticity: The physiological basis of rehabilitation.* 2nd ed. Philadelphia: Lippincot Williams & Wilkins.

Logan, G.A., and W.C. McKinney. 1970. *Kinesiology.* Dubuque, IA: Brown.

Loy, S.F., J.J. Hoffmann, and G.J. Holland. 1995. Benefits and practical use of cross-training in sports. *Sports Medicine* 19 (1): 1-8.

Maglischo, E.W. 2003. *Swimming fastest.* Champaign, IL: Human Kinetics.

McArdle, W.D., F.I. Katch, and V.L. Katch. 2001. *Exercise physiology: Energy, nutrition and human performance.* 5th ed. Baltimore: Williams & Wilkins.

McClay, I.S., J.R. Robinson, T.P. Andriacci, et al. 1994a. A kinematic profile of skills in professional basketball players. *Journal of Applied Biomechanics* 10 (3): 205-221.

McClay, I.S., J.R. Robinson, T.P. Andriacci, et al. 1994b. A profile of ground reaction forces in professional basketball. *Journal of Applied Biomechanics* 10 (3): 221-236.

McGill, S. 2002. *Low back disorders.* Champaign, IL: Human Kinetics.

McGrath, M. 2001. Designer movement: Movement and function. Principles of the human body. Presentation at UK Coaches Institute Conference, Cardiff, Wales.

McInnes, S.E., J.S. Carlson, C.J. Jones, and M.J. McKenna. 1995. The physiological load imposed on basketball players during competition. *Journal of Sports Sciences* 13:387-397.

Mujika, I., and S. Padilla. 2003. Scientific bases for precompetition tapering strategies. *Medicine & Science in Sports & Exercise* 35 (7): 1182-1187.

Mulak, J. 1964. Mihaly Igloi's Training Method. Chap. 8 in *Run, run, run.* Fred Wilt. Los Altos, CA: Tafnews Press.

Olbrecht, J. 2000. *The science of winning: Planning, periodizing and optimizing swim training.* Luton, UK: Swimshop.

Oschman, J.L. 2003. *Energy medicine in therapeutics and human performance.* Amsterdam: Butterworth Heinemann.

Radcliffe, J.C., and R.C. Farentinos. 1999. *High-powered plyometrics.* Champaign, IL: Human Kinetics.

Robertson, S., and R. Way. 2005. Long-term athlete development: A made in Canada model. *Coaches Report* 11 (3): 7.

Sale, D. 1986. Neural adaptation in strength and power training. In *Human muscle power*, ed. N.L. Jones. Champaign, IL: Human Kinetics.

Shrier, I. 1999. Stretching before exercise does not reduce the risk of local muscle injury: A critical review of the clinical and basic science literature. *Clinical Journal of Sport Medicine* Oct 9 (4): P221-227.

Thacker, S.B., J. Gilchrist, D.F. Stroup, and C.D. Kimsey Jr. 2004. The impact of stretching on sports injury risk: A systematic review of the literature. *Medicine & Science in Sports & Exercise* 36 (4): 371-378.

Todd, M.E. 1937. *The thinking body.* Highston, NJ: Princeton Books.

Wilson, G.J. 1994. Strength and power in sport. In *Applied anatomy and biomechanics in sport* by J. Bloomfield, T.R. Ackland, and B.C. Elliot. Carlton, Australia: Blackwell.

Wilson, G.J., R.U. Newton, A.J. Murphy, and B.J. Humphries. 1993. The optimal training load for the development of dynamic athletic performance. *Medicine & Science in Sports & Exercise* 23: 1279-1286.

Young, W.B., M.H. McDowell, and B.J. Scarlett. 2001. Specificity of sprint and agility training methods. *Journal of Strength and Conditioning Research* 15 (3): 315-319.

Zatsiorsky, V.M. 1995. *Science and practice of strength training.* Champaign, IL: Human Kinetics.

Index

Note: The italicized *f* and *t* following page numbers refer to figures and table, respectively.

About the Author

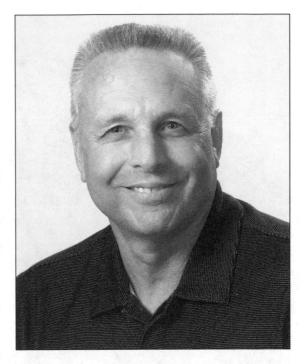

Vern Gambetta is currently the director of Gambetta Sports Training Systems. He served as the director of athletic development for the New York Mets (2004-2005), speed and conditioning coach for the Tampa Bay Mutiny major league soccer team (1996, 1997, and 1999), conditioning consultant to the U.S. men's 1998 World Cup soccer team and the New England Revolution (1998), and director of conditioning for the Chicago White Sox. Gambetta has also worked with the Canadian men's and women's national basketball teams and the Chicago Bulls. He was also one of the founders and the first director of the USA Track & Field Coaching Education program. Recognized internationally as an expert in training and conditioning for sport, Gambetta has lectured extensively and conducted clinics in Canada, Japan, Australia, and Europe. For more information, visit www.gambetta.com.

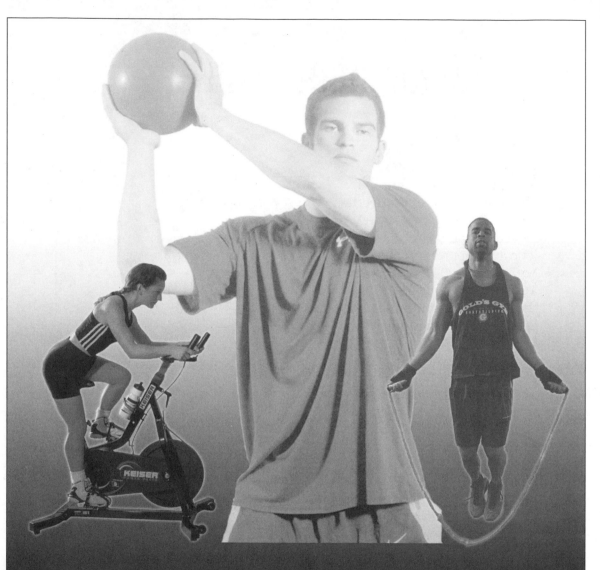

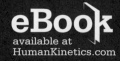